Crystal Healing

Charge Up Your Mind Body and Soul Beginner's Journey

(Transform Your Life With the Healing Power of Crystals)

John Waits

Published By **Chris David**

John Waits

All Rights Reserved

Crystal Healing: Charge Up Your Mind Body and Soul Beginner's Journey (Transform Your Life With the Healing Power of Crystals)

ISBN 978-1-77485-992-6

No part of this guidebook shall be reproduced in any form without permission in writing from the publisher except in the case of brief quotations embodied in critical articles or reviews.

Legal & Disclaimer

The information contained in this ebook is not designed to replace or take the place of any form of medicine or professional medical advice. The information in this ebook has been provided for educational & entertainment purposes only.

The information contained in this book has been compiled from sources deemed reliable, and it is accurate to the best of the Author's knowledge; however, the Author cannot guarantee its accuracy and validity and cannot be held liable for any errors or omissions. Changes are periodically made to this book. You must consult your doctor or get professional medical advice before using any of the suggested remedies, techniques, or information in this book.

Upon using the information contained in this book, you agree to hold harmless the Author from and against any damages, costs, and expenses, including any legal fees potentially resulting from the application of any of the information provided by this guide. This disclaimer applies to any damages or injury caused by the use and application, whether directly or indirectly, of any advice or information presented, whether for breach of contract, tort, negligence, personal injury, criminal intent, or under any other cause of action.

You agree to accept all risks of using the information presented inside this book. You need to consult a professional medical practitioner in order to ensure you are both able and healthy enough to participate in this program.

Table Of Contents

Chapter 1: Crystal Healing And Your Well-Being 1

Chapter 2: Crystal Healing And Bruxism . 23

Chapter 3: Mental Health 55

Chapter 4: Crystal Therapy: Updated 83

Chapter 5: Healing Gemstones & Crystals: Inspiring Well-Being And Balance 109

Chapter 6: Seven Chakras Overview 137

Chapter 7: How To Choose Your Crystals 148

Chapter 8: Crystals 166

Chapter 9: Uses For Crystals 181

Chapter 1: Crystal Healing And Your Well-Being
F

Crystals have been treasured for their healing properties or beauty. To display various crystals and describe their geological roots, the Melbourne Art Gallery has built several rooms. Another similar exhibit can be found in the Museum at Bathurst in NSW. Over the years, skepticals have been dismissive about crystal healing. This is why it is so refreshing to see them dedicate several rooms to these museums.

There are many books available that discuss the benefits of crystal healing.

We will go back to school's science laboratory for an explanation. We discovered that all things are made of atoms. Solids are composed many small particles which move and appear reliable because the grains of solid are so dense (closed-together) that they seem solid. Denser liquids containing atoms of different sizes are liquids. Less solid liquids are gas. Like you and I, everything around us is composed of atoms or even small particles that oscillate. But our senses don't pick them up so we don't see them move. These atoms are also composed of crystals which, at a particular rate, oscillate or move. UCLA has performed experiments to understand this over the last 50 years. They can also be found on the Internet.

You are unique in how you travel, think and feel. There is no other person in this world that you can clone. People's vibrations can influence us. You've probably spent an hour listening and then putting the phone down. We are constantly capturing the " vibes" of others, and encouraging them to connect with us. Also, crystals and other objects around us emit a particular vibration, which can be used to distinguish rose quartz crystals from those made of topaz.

Crystals are unique in that each crystal has a different geometrial arrangement and oscillates (vibrate), thus making them distinct by name. The smokey quartz is distinct from the amethyst which works in close contact with us. Because the crystal is nearby us, our vibrations change. This is the same research that was previously made available on the Internet. As they interact directly with our vibrations, energy centers, and alter the way atoms oscillate, they are thought to have a positive impact on us. The books that detail the different attributes of each crystal will reveal how they affect you. You'll also learn about how each crystal can treat various emotions. Many people report feeling different after receiving a healing from a crystal. Even though many people believe otherwise there must be an explanation for why people believe differently. It is clear that this could not be just a placebo effect.

The healer may place crystals around or on the body of the customer during crystal healing. The patient will usually lie on the ground or in a chair. It is best to have a dimmed room with a soothing scent of candles or incense, as well as soft music. The purpose of the massage is to help the patient relax and complete the job. The healing required will dictate the length of time.

Crystals, it is believed, alter how the energy centres of the body (chakras), vibrate. They also stabilize and reverse mental or emotional barriers in both mind and physical bodies. By removing these blocks, new energy can reach the people and help them to improve their lives, health, and provide more resources.

Crystals can therefore be used to soothe and heal the body, mind as well as emotions and spirit. Your personal experience will determine whether it is right for your needs. It is best to try it yourself. It is not possible for one or two healings only to make miracles. It took you many months, or even years, of neglect in various areas of your lives to get your bag and disease here. And there is no magic wand to cure it. This is life. It's not TV. But healing takes time.

Healing at Home

Home healing is possible for anyone. You have many options. Not all of them are perfect. Here are some suggestions to help you start your journey to healing. These are easy steps that nearly everyone can take after reading the book.

Affirmation Therapy: It is easy and very straightforward to use. Use positive affirmations to transform your subconscious programming into positive attitudes. It takes around 21 days for this to happen, but that's just one drop in the bucket when you consider the whole picture. Use constructive language and focus on your comments. When you put your attention on others' love, you might claim that you are worthy of it. It is about making the most of it now and shaping it positively. Repeat this process every day for 21 consecutive days (3 times per day).

Prayer Healing: Prayers can be used to heal yourself by increasing the energy and flow of your healing work. You think that is enough? It is a mixture of prayer and work to heal a particular problem in your own life. Prayer-healing is possible in a quiet place twice per day (morning, and night). It is not as fast or easy as prayer healing. Here is an example from a Financial Priest that will help you formulate a healing Prayer: Financial Healing prayer: I ask you for guidance and healing during the meditation/prayer. I appeal to the Universe / Divine Soul / Ascended Master/God/Angel to assist me in solving all my financial problems and provide healing energy. I am open and willing to work with anyone who holds me back or helps me heal any areas. These are my issues. I am open to positive energy in the financial and money areas of my life.

Crystal Healing is the art of using crystal vibrations and their healing properties to heal. If you want to increase your energy flow for your home and office, you can make an Emerald gemstone elixir by adding water. This will dampen the surrounding environment twice daily, so that it changes the energy flow vibrationally. Crystal healing will solve all your energy, psychological, cognitive, and spiritual problems. As many crystals have the ability to assist with crystal healing, this means that you can identify what is causing your problem. You will notice that some crystals have a greater effect on your vibrational frequencies than others. It is up to you to discover the one that resonates with your energy fields. The best place to start is with the Emeralds.

Energy cure: Energy therapy is about managing the flow of energy, eliminating any issues, creating positive healing energy, improving a person's vibration, and increasing their energy make up. You can even learn how to use other energy formats. Usui Reiki, a broad Reiki healing technique that many people use to their healing powers, is easy. Additionally, you can work with energy modalities that are more in tune to your vibrational healing speeds, such energy control formats, for healing protection, etc. Energy healing involves treating the root cause, not only the symptoms. Then, we balance the power flow and cure the problem.

There are many other healing methods. I'm only listing a few. Learn more about angelic and natural healing, healing from the divine sources, herbal healing, color therapy, and other healing methods. It's all about finding your energy and what you feel is most beneficial for you. This is how we balance our emotional energy fields!

A Crystal Healing

Energy and Protection Energy and information all form part of the physical universe. While energy vibrates at different frequencies we can't see it because it vibrates so fast that our senses cannot pick up on it. Our senses are too slow to detect these vibrations. We receive information that helps us see the chair in which we sit, as well as our bodies and those of others.

If you walk into a room feeling like you can "cut through the atmosphere with your knife", that is called negative energy.

Also, positive and negative energy can be drawn from opening our centers of energy for healing, meditation or visualization. It is important to protect yourself against negative energy.

Grounding is important before you work with your crystals. It keeps you in touch with your earthly world. Working with crystals after you've completed your work will take you up to a higher stage. You may feel like floating, or emotional, and you could feel like you're on a healing curve.

Take three deep breaths, lie down with your feet flat on the floor, and you will feel the roots reaching from your feet. These roots will reach the earth's core, the soil, and through the wall. To test your grounding you can lift your feet off the floor. It is easy to tell if it is difficult.

Dear Heaven, I ask for your pure white light to surround me. Please remove me from all the harmful vibrations of the universe, without causing harm to any living thing. Please surround me with your total protection golden bubble.

Visualization Visualize your self in a pink bubble. It will help you to see that nothing but divine white light is available and unconditional love can penetrate it.

White is the color of eternal security. Red is the color of unconditional love.

The crystals can be cleaned and blessed in many different ways. Crystals cannot be placed in water. It is important to ensure that your crystals are properly cleaned.

Manual cleaning is not necessary as experiences can create crystals. If you have crystals from other sources, you'll need to wash them.

Use a child's brush to clean crystals.

Crystals must first be blessed before use. This prayer should be said after the crystal has been thoroughly cleaned.

Mother Earth is a wonderful source of crystals that I am grateful for. I request that the crystals be blessed in order to release all negative energies into the world, without affecting those living.

Working with crystals

* Make sure to follow the steps before working with crystals.

* Protect yourself and keep your ground!

* Cleanse crystal and bend it

* With your eyes closed, sit down and focus for a while.

You can hold the single crystal in your right hand, pointing any point toward your fingers.

Use your left hand to hold the crystal. Point the point at your site and ask for assistance. Each side should be used for at least 10 mins.

You should enjoy your new crystal. It will become apparent that you are sensitive to his field.

* Step 1. Look at the crystal in different angles. Then, close your eyes. Take out your notes and hold it in your hands.

* Step 2 Place the crystal in your palms and imagine the air moving through it. Next, take a deep breath and exhale through the crystal. This will create energy.

Step 3: With your eyes closed, sit quietly and focus on the palm color. You can feel any vibrations and thoughts.

* Step 4. Sit down on your solarplexus and feel it. Once again, picture the crystal's color and form.

You will notice any changes in your third eye if you do it again.

Crystals are a powerful healing tool

Crystal healing involves the use crystals to improve and transform skin, body, or mind. It helped me heal from emotional trauma. I have found that crystals have made a significant difference in my life, both energetically and physically. Both gemstones can be used to alter your vibrational frequency. You can alter your vibrational frequency simply by placing either gemstones or auras on your body. They can also be used to amplify your goal. You can achieve the desired outcome faster by improving your objective.

There are many kinds of crystals. They come in different sizes, colors, and types. Each crystal has its own unique properties and can be used to solve various problems. But you won't be able to study the crystals that you desire and search for them. The crystals will select you if you do it the other way around. If you're at a crystal pick shop, stop and find the crystal that interests you.

There are several things you need to do before your new natural goods can be prepared. These next steps are necessary for crystal healing. I know you are very excited about it and are eager to use it immediately.

First, clean the crystals of any negative energy. If they were in the supermarket, they might have been approached by several people, who could have easily absorbed their negativity. You don't want this in your energy field. It is important to wash your crystals regularly depending on how often you use them. There are several crystal clearing methods that can be used. To clear all negative energy, the easiest and most effective method is to put it in your mouth. Then, run water under it for about one to two minutes. The hull will work fine. The hull can be cleaned in several ways. Step two involves aligning the crystal to the current vibrational frequency. Hold the crystal with your fingers and close your eyes. You can either say it aloud or feel it important in any other way. You will mount your crystals in phase 3. Put your crystals out in direct sunlight for no less than 5 hours. You can also put them in the shade of a new or full moon overnight. Plan how you'll use your crystals. You could argue that the crystals can be used to heal, protect, or ground. This is an optional choice that can or cannot happen. Programming a crystal in a specific application will allow you to adjust it to the sound of what you want. You can hold the crystal in one hand, and then say, "This crystal has been used in your hands. Fill it with white." You can repeat these words up to four more times to configure the crystal. You can now use your new glasses.

Your needs will dictate how you use your crystals. These crystals may be worn as jewels, or you can carry one or two of them in your bag. Please remember to clean the crystals more often, as they can absorb harmful rays from your environment. You can meditate on or around crystals to improve your meditation. Place the crystals that correspond to your

Chakras on each chakra and you will be able to balance them. Crystals can also be held in your office or room for security or clearing. You could even place stones under the pillow in the night to improve your dreams and help you remember them. Crystals have many benefits that will improve your life in every area.

Crystals are used for many purposes... For the past 30+ years, people have used crystals for their medicinal purposes.

* How you can alter the energy in crystals in an area you live or work

* You can also create crystal patterns with a specific vibration

* The clearing procedure for crystals

* When to use what crystals...

* What to avoid using your amethyst quartz Purifies Water Amethyst Crystal discovered that the amethyst is more effective than a water purifier. Our water was purified using tiny amethyst pieces in the water jug instead of a water purification machine.

Alchemy has occurred, with all the chlorine, the taste, coming from unpurified (unpleasant), tap water... Water was drained, then it was delicious to drink.

Now take a crystal and place it in your hand. Imagine the perfect vibration that would descend from the heavens through the physical body of the crystal's owner and enable it to transmit the vibration to the crystal.

Significantly, a customer lived in a place of panic and overwhelming. She believed that she would feel invaded.

When she walked in front of her front door, she felt the vibration. Her handbag would be far away from her and she would feel the security.

Crystal Empowered Changed

It is a way of life. The way you feel can be changed by vibrationally opening or closing a crystal you are in love with. Do it now. Try it today.

She felt the overwhelming pressure to contact her doctor immediately she opened the packet and held the crystal. This result has completely blown her away.

She had an intuitive feeling and rectal carcinoma was found. The hospital couldn't have done anything for her, and she would've lived a much longer life if she had not been there.

This is the power these amazing transmitters have. And... And... It's amazing how much you will love the results of crystals if your ability to experiment with them and to become immune to them.

Don't fall asleep with crystals.

Avoid putting crystals in your room. Crystal chatting is what we refer to as affecting your sleep quality. Some said that their crystals kept people awake through the night. It was reported that their crystals caused them to have disturbing, but still strong, dreams. Perhaps their soul, mind, or body were not allowed rest.

It's called crystal power. It's the crystal power. Take them out, get rid of the energy and then move them to another part of the room. It'll surprise you how much this will improve your night.

Crystal Healing - Alternative Natural Therapy

Crystal Healers

For thousands of years crystal healers were used to provide alternative healing or holistic therapy. Crystal healers with the aura and authority of an authority use various patterns of natural crystals that allow them to treat physical conditions as well as mental ones. Gemstone therapy is also known as crystal healing. The methods used by crystal healers are as varied as their crystals.

Crystal healers are able to heal the body and mind by using crystals to stimulate the chakras. A chakra refers all to the spiritual energy. Each of the seven chakras within the body form the power of a person. If one chakra is out of balance, it can bring about negative or harmful energies into the body. The precious gemstones channel the positive energy to the body and redirect the negative vitality. They also restore the equilibrium that the chakras naturally have. These crystals are used to heal psychological misdirection, health disorders, and other issues.

The legend of the crystal healers is found in almost every culture, from the Indian tribes all the way to the Egyptians. Although the originator of the use a crystal for mental and physical therapy remains elusive, it has been proven that this method is still widely used in the world today. Jade amulets are believed to help guide the soul to its final destination. Even King Tut's grave was covered in jade amulets. Chinese culture still strongly believes in the use crystal healers, primarily jade, emerald, that are supposed to improve their intelligence and memory. Kristal healers can use lapidarylazuli, amethyst, agate and all kinds of amulets in order to ease stress.

Crystal Healers' Benefits

This can bring about a variety of benefits that will enhance the spiritual and bodily characteristics of an individual. Some of the most important benefits of crystal healing include self-improvement, vitality, and health.

When conventional medicine is failing to work, healers can help you. You can use a crystal remedy to reduce stress, anxiety, and depression. It can be used to treat digestive problems, pain relief, headaches, sleep problems, migraines, stomach problems, stress, and anxiety. It has demonstrated excellent results in friendship, asset creation, self-realization, and personal self realization.

Crystal therapy is a natural way to heal the body. It involves deep relaxation and meditation. It balances the mind, spirit and body. It can enhance imagination, increase communication, and allow you to grow your spirituality. Although it is not meant to replace medical attention, it can help you feel better and make your mind and body stronger. The many benefits that healers can offer include increased pride, love, and relief of migraines.

What is Crystal Healing?

You can do it with a crystal healing practitioner. They place crystals all over the body. The energy grid is used to remove negative energy and create the right energy. Crystal healers surround people with healing energy. This helps to clear the aura of blocked chakras. You can use the same color crystals as the chakra to provide healing vibrations. It creates positive waves that attract positive things in the life of those who use a healer.

Crystal healers are usually found in tranquility or comfort areas. The healer is fully dressed and asks what you feel is wrong to determine whether crystals should be used to unblock the chakras. Amber, rose lepidolite (and stability) are some of the most used gems for healing. Each of them offers another healing asset. Amber, for example helps you love yourself and boost your self-esteem. Selenite helps you access the energy of your higher consciousness. It is possible to heal oneself from within with crystal healers. The workshops of crystal healers provide a broad overview of crystal healing and the ways it can transform a person's life. A person can learn relaxation techniques and visualization to balance the chakras and remove negative energy from the body during the workshops of a crystal healer.

Chapter 2: Crystal Healing And Bruxism

Bruxism refers to teeth grinding. These effects can affect both adults and children.

There is no one answer. Some believe Bruxism can be attributed a lack in tooth coordination. Others think it may be due to depression, a digestive disorder, sleep disturbance, or a central nervous disorder.

It is affected by reflex chewing. This is because chewing is not an acquired habit. The mechanical brain is activated when a person goes to sleep, while the brain control stays inactive. This causes Bruxism (an irregular chewing activity).

Bruxism occurs when you are sleeping, even if it is for a brief time.

The typical case is where the incisors press laterally against the canines. This damages the enamel. It can result in biting by removing sharp edges or flattening teeth. It is the most prevalent sleep disorder, with 30-40 million Americans being active at night.

Bruxism can lead to extreme stress levels. The pressure on the teeth during an episode ranges between 100 and 600 psi (pounds/square-inch). While everyone does this, others may do it differently and may not think about extreme cases.

Bruxism may cause problems such as jaw headaches or teeth already decayed (from another source), tooth loss, cavities, irritations, and heavy cheek and temple muscles. Teeth that become susceptible to gum infection, shrinking of teeth, and tooth splits are all possible.

Below are two healing crystals that will help you with your problem. It is best to place them under your bed or beside your bed. The crystals can be used while you sleep, so you don't have need to hold them constantly. You should program crystals to assist with Bruxism Healing before you use them.

Gehlenite enhances optimism. The practical side of your nature stimulates circulation.

Stromboli - Bringing love and generosity into the ground. This enhances peace, happiness and harmony.

It is wonderful to transfer energy between the healer and the recipient.

Not all crystals are created equal.

You can use these crystals to help explain why grinding is bad.

Fluorite is likely the next best choice crystal to treat any type of teeth problem. This crystal is highly protective and can be used to clean up long-standing behavioral patterns. Fluorite is an excellent crystal to study because it helps students organize and process data and allows them to recall what they have learned. Fluorite is a great way to increase your intuition, and fight geometric and geopathic tension. This has an impartial, stabilizing effect on emotions. It can treat allergies, ulcers, rheumatism, and other conditions.

Stress is another reason that makes the disease more serious. Hematite: The brain, which can be used to obtain a great legal outcome, helps body, mind, and body are harmonised. Women, especially those who are shy and sensitive, will benefit from crystals' healing powers. It's a good crystal to ground yourself and reduce stress. It improves self-esteem, balances meridians, protects, and is a great choice for anyone looking to boost their confidence. This crystal is great for learning mathematics and enhancing power. Hematite aids in transcending autonomous limitations and restrictions. It also strengthens our instincts for survival. Arthritis and blood conditions are some of the ailments that support crystal healing properties.

Amethysts: A powerful, healing, and protective crystal, they are especially strong. This helps to reduce spiritual attacks and insomnia. A brain that is not asleep improves memory and relies on frustration, fear, and anxiety. Stress encourages love and is useful in screening for meditational disorders that support amethyst-healing.

The three crystals listed above should always be kept with you. You can wear them as jewelry, or keep them in your pocket or purse in the form of a rock of worry or a pawn rock.

Also, clean and program your crystals for stress relief.

How to Use Quartz Healing Stones

What is crystal Aura and healing? They are crystals. A pair of Clear Quartz crystals can detoxify and restore your physical, spiritual and psychological Aura and the Ether energy field. They can be used as a single crystal or in combination with other crystals or minerals.

What are the crystals doing here? These crystals enable the user to channel pure divine energy into their body. Glasses can be used to increase the body's ability to heal itself and to absorb energy at higher frequencies.

Clear Quartz Healing Stones cannot be used during cure sessions unless you choose to allow them to choose you. It is best to test the vibration of the crystals before you can determine which ones are correct.

If you happen to have crystals that are already found in pairs, you can rest assured that most of the work has been done for you. Simply "press" on the crystals you like. How would you know which ones are right for your? Calm down and breathe deeply. Now, slowly move your left arm over each set. Your power and the crystals that radiate heat/distinctive energy into each set resonate best with your power.

You can use the crystals to verify what you are hearing or feeling. The crystal point should always be guided towards your wrist in your lefthand. The end crystal in your right handed hand should go back from your wrist to you hands.

So that energy flows through your body, it is essential that the quartz healing Crystals be held in both of your hands. If you hold the set of healing crystals in your hands, you are a conduit for Divine Energy. You can allow the energy to flow into and out of your body.

You will need to decide which crystals you'd like to use. Before using crystals, clean them. Your crystals can be purified and recharged by running them under freshwater.

You can begin using the healing stones. Your mind will be quiet. Keep the gems in your mouth and exhale slowly three times. You can speak aloud to yourself or silently. Spark is what I invoke, and if God is in me, I am a pure and flawless source of Light.

A gentle, tingling sensation can initially be felt. It may take some practice before you can sense and feel energy flowing through crystals. It does not matter if the crystals flow into you immediately or not. Trust it.

The healing crystal located in your left-hand draws pure Divine Source energies. The power flowing through your right hand is enough to take all that isn't necessary. You can also open your heart to Divine Origin and allow Divine White Light and all of the negative energy to flow through you.

You should be aware that your aura is a reflection on what is happening in your physical body.

This is an easy self-healing way to heal yourself. You simply need to sit down in a mediating chair, then stand straight up with your neck extended.

You can choose whether to spend 10 minutes or 15 minutes the first time you try this crystal healing method. You will begin to notice changes in your body as you become more confident and feel at ease. You will start to feel harmony, peace, and more frequent observation.

Wash the crystals after the session. Your inner detoxification and healing process will be completed by increasing your water intake in the next 24hrs.

This simple technique for crystal healing is highly effective. You will experience a greater sense of well-being and a better quality of life by working with crystals.

Crystal Healing Scientific Evidence

Crystal Healing proponents are around for decades. It is sometimes believed to be deceit. The theoretical mechanism that allows our body transmissions from radiating stones was discovered during a research project.

It's not quackery. Crystal Healing.

The third eyes The third eye is the oldest of our ancestors. It was able to absorb external movements, such as light of various frequencies. It has grown to become our pineal gidd over the years. It now secretes the hormone melatonin, which is vital for every day of our lives.

The research shows how the body absorbs external vibrations.

Amethyst crystalline had the best measured energy field. It also had the most data from all of the types of crystals examined. This was why most of our evaluations were performed on amethyst crystal.

The Einstein equation $E=MC2$, which demonstrates that our bodies must be two matrices, one made of matter (M) as well as one made of energy (E), is a great guide for science understanding. Crystal Healing supporters call this electromagnetic fields their aura. (c stands for the speed of light.

The primary goal of the research then was to find a mechanism that would allow our bodies receive energy from a radiating stone. These are where Chakras, auras, and energy come into play.

Chakras Chakra is an old Sanskrit name for "wheel" (or "circle") and it is used to refer to seven specific energy centers along a meridian. Brow Chakra refers to the Third Eye and is one the most important research tools.

Western philosophy views Chakras generally as ancient myths, which is a baseless assumption.

Many Americans dismiss the idea of Chakras being "new-age" ideas. However, the idea of the chakra goes back thousands of years.

The Vedas described the first Chakras in the Vedas. Thus, the Hindu scriptures were established. The evidence indicates that the Vedas were brought into India from prehistoric

India by the early founders, who came from a lost civilization. Plato believed that Atlantis is a society.

Chakras, located in the physical body, are thought to be "force centers", occupied by whorls o energy. They can also be found in the physical body at these stages.

Many people believe the chakras to be symbolic. To fully understand the physical nature of chakras, and their role as energy disks, it is important not to forget that energy is also physical. It is heat that powers our nervous and brainwave systems.

The Brow Chakra (also known as the Third Eye) is the most significant in Crystal Healing. The Third Eye is a reminder that our ancient ancestors were able to detect vibrations from the environment. Many wild creatures such as the Mantis, Iguana and other Iguanas have third ears.

Crystal Healing is described by its advocates as a powerful, profound and gentle healing technique. This software concentrates energy from different crystals to the Chakras, Aura Fields, and Chakras. The energy is directed to the Chakras and Aura points that are most sensitive.

They claim that the energy flows through our Chakras and Auras to all areas of our lives.

Each chakra has its own significance as they each involve an endocrine hormone.

Auras Auras are the electromagnetic fields that surround the human body and all other organisms. This is a proven scientific fact.

Crystal Healing devotees maintain that an aura can reveal if someone communicates with another entity or is religious. These devotees believe that the characters of an individual can reveal their well-being. They believe that aura colors are a sign of certain characteristics. You should remember that every color is a different frequency or vibration spectrum.

Intelligence can be indicated by Ruby Red and Violet. It also indicates vitality. Violet is associated with love and healing. Gray can indicate fear and Gray can indicate cruelty and stubbornness.

Evidence has shown that our third eye (our pinealglass) can sense the energy of crystals with perfect or close to perfect properties.

To understand how it works, you must realize that our bodies can be thought of as energy matrices. Additionally, amethyst and amethyst Crystals can be energy matrices.

Let's look at how the vibration of energy in a crystal interacts to the power of the human electromagnetic field. The uniform crystal vibrations tend to calmen the atmosphere.

This is what crystal cure is all about.

Research has led to the discovery of the theoretical mechanism by which radiant crystals can be transferred to the body's energy fields.

Our Third Eye, an ancient eye, evolved in a way that can absorb external signals. This includes frequencies of individual crystals.

Third Eye Development, crystal healing & psychic ability

Learn more about crystal healing. It is revealed that your third-eye can use a higher dimension. These techniques include visualizations and exercises that direct the energies of the inner system to activate your third eye.

Through the creation of a third eye, your intuition can also be developed. As you become more aware, your awareness, perception, astral plane memory and experience will improve. You will notice a greater activation of your third eye through practice. This will allow for more intuition flashes. She explains how we can focus our minds on the midpoint between the pineal and pituitary bodies to create a magnetic force that allows us to picture something. This also helps the mind to have energy that gives life and direction. How to use a pendulum from crystal

Although we can all see shapes or images with our eyes closed, few people can fully grasp the meaning of these images. The book will teach how to see your higher self, spiritual guides and other spirit mates.

Most rituals and religious traditions can see with the help of higher energy field knowledge in the third eye.

The third eye can be used to gain specific soul layers or dimensions. The soul can also be referred to as time, the past and the present. Most people describe it as having recollections. The third eye allows us the ability to travel into another dimension. Many people have experienced this partly through dreams or visions. Our ability to adjust our third eye allows us to have greater flexibility and clarity.

The third eye can be affected by moods, medication, food, drinks, and even medications. Over-stimulated people will often have their third eyes closed. The possibility of sensory overload can be caused by excessive use of radio or television. This can cause stress to the body and alter the soul's interaction.

The techniques described here will help you create the impression that your third eye feels like it is floating on energy. Note: This operation does not create third eye sight, but rather the impression that your third eye has a focus and attention that allows you to balance and coordinate your performance. The third eye is responsible in selection, individuality, imagination.

Lynn's straightforward writing style allows us all to follow more complex topics, such as * making crystals using and the energy within them and how to feed it; * general curing with crystals, which includes treatment with colors, chakras and auras.

Crystal Healing is jam-packed of information. The information is comprehensive and easy to understand. This book will teach you everything you need for a career as a crystal healing practitioner. This book will teach you how to heal yourself, make friends and start your own therapy practice.

Try it. Try it.

You can relax in a quiet area and clear your mind. After taking a few deep, slow breaths, focus your attention on your screen.

You should be able to recognize colors. Relax and take deep, slow breaths. You will see the colors transform into shapes. If you keep your eyes on the colors, you may recognize the shape.

If you don't see anything, go back later and try again.

This book will show you how to recognize your emotions, energy centers and thoughts. You will be able to transform your entire life. You will discover how being disconnected from your emotions leads to insecurity and vulnerability.

Lynn will show you how mindfulness and relaxation can help you find inner peace and harmony. Your everyday life will be easier, you'll be able to reduce stress and tackle your problems. This experience can change your life.

She will show how to believe in your instincts and insight, as well as how to use the third eye, your eyesight. When you trust your judgement, you make accurate decisions.

Balancing your chakras is a way to regulate energy flow. You can detect and see the energy colors in the body and read the auras.

How can you relieve stress and pain? By manipulating the power and strength of the bodies to support others.

Understanding dream perception and sleep is a way to see the subconscious. This is an important aspect, as you can learn and be told a lot from your sleep. This is how your dreams are controlled and how astral voyages and astral planes help you get to the spiritual world.

You can use mental tools such as Clairvoyant vision or Tarot Cards to predict the future.

You'll learn how to connect with your chosen spirit -- understanding messages from the religious world, talking, listening, and contacting your spiritual guide.

Reiki and Crystals

Once you have understood the principles of Reiki, you will be able to study crystals and determine if they are a good fit for you.

Crystals may be placed on or in the aura. They can also be used to purify the home, to absorb energy from your computer or to absorb radiation.

You can strategically place crystals throughout your home to counter geopathic pressures and protect the environment. The gems can also be worn as jewelry or carried in the pocket. To purify and strengthen them, you can also put crystals into your potable water bottle.

Place a foundationstone such as smoky Quartz or hematite in the earth Chakra just below your feet. This is done at the beginning of every healing process, as the stones assist in the removal of negative energy. Because these stones are often a recipient of negative or unwanted energy, it is essential that you purify them after each treatment.

Multiple crystals can be used to effectually activate each of the chakras. Just a handful of these healing stones have been included to show you the range of options available. Smoky quartz can be used to purify and soil the root chakra. You can also opt for a crystal-like, red carnelian. This is a stabilizing stone which encourages self-confidence. Red jasper stimulates energy and can also help to heal the circulatory, digestive and sexual organs.

If you have a patient with a specific problem to heal, choose crystals based on their healing abilities. Please remember to rinse your healing crystals with water after every use. It can be rinsed with saltwater or run it under water. You can also hold them in your hands to purify and strengthen the power. You can visualize the symbols Cho Ku Rei, Sei He Ki which penetrate every stone with Reiki 2. Finally, you have the option to put your crystals in sunlight to absorb more of the sun's energy.

For the sacred chakra, use red jasper to heal your sexual organs. Orange Calcite helps you to overcome depression, balance emotions, and remove fear. Bowel disease, which affects the reproductive system, gallbladder or intestinal, is treated.

You can learn the qualities of every pier through a crystal guide. Find the stones that resonate best with you, and include them in any healing. Let your intuition choose the stone for each of your healings most often. If necessary, excuse yourself from laziness and let your hand hover on the healing crystals until it feels natural to pick a few to give to the patient.

Yellow tourmaline activates solar plexus and increases personal strength. The physical treatment includes the stomach, liver, gallbladder (spleen), stomach, liver, kidneys and spleen. Another wonderful stone is called the "eye of the Tiger". It works to increase self-worth and express willpower. For use on the chakras in the solar plexus, most crystals have a yellow or golden color.

If you are beginning a healing process, you will be able to detect any blockages or weaknesses in the chakras. The crystal can be placed directly on the chakra to aid in healing. The crystal acts as your third hand during healing.

Most people report feeling handed over to their chakras after moving to another healing spot.

Rose quartz stands for unconditional love. It purifies and enchants the heart, on all levels. If you are able to strengthen your self-love you will attract loving relationships in your life.

Rhodonite, another pink-colored stone, can be found just above or directly below the heart chakra. Rhodonite is a stone that can heal emotional injuries and help to transform difficult emotions. It can be used to efficiently work with the heart in green like green quartz, green tourmaline or moose agate.

It will make your throat ache if you directly place a crystal on it. It is preferable to place your chosen glasses on either one side or under your mouth. Blue quartz is usually used. It was obtained in Capilla del Monte (a magical town in Central Argentina). It can be used to heal throat issues. This stone was a personal favorite of mine for a while, so I kept it in the pocket. As standard (and attuned me). This shows that having faith in a healing crystal and regular contact with them helps you to treat better.

Lapis Lazuli regulates and treats the throat chakra. It also treats the stomach, thyroid, stomach, and thymus. The important challenges that the throat chakra presents are thought to help with self-awareness as well as self-expression. Lapis jewelry is beautiful and can be worn to enhance your chest.

Lapis Lazuli is a good choice for the brow chakra. It can promote illumination, improve intuition abilities, and guide your spiritual journey. Purple amethyst works well when you are meditating, healing yourself, or helping others. His healing work was done with amethyst over many years. This stone was his gift to me. Amethyst carries an energetic vibration that is good for the soul. It increases common sense, spiritual understandings, intuition, and mental abilities. You can use it on your brow chakra.

The crown chakra is also aided by violet amethyst, which helps to strengthen the mental, physical, and spiritual connections. The aura can be purified and negative energy transformed. It is one the most spiritual pillars.

A gem shop can help you find the right stones for your needs. Keep any stone you like and hold it in your hand. If you find it appealing, it might just be your rock. The dealer can help you to discuss the stone properties and their healing and other esoteric characteristics. You'll discover the crystals that suit you best using intuition, experience, and touch. You can also take your pendulum to a gem shop to see which crystals match your energy.

As a final reminder, crystals come in many shapes, sizes, and processing. Although you will find polished stones that create beautiful slopes, I believe this process distracts from the pure beauty of the natural stone. The earth is unpolished. Crystals can be artistically shaped into shapes such as walls, circles or hearts. Round crystals can pose a problem. They did not breathe genuinely until the glass rolled onto its head and fell to the ground, rolling all over the room.

Natural Healing Methods: A Guide

This guide will help you to heal yourself naturally using natural healing methods.

Natural healing does not have to be difficult or complicated. While it might take some education to learn how to use natural healing, once you have read this chapter you will be able to still benefit from some form of it.

Let's start by defining natural healing methods. These include acupressure (homeopathy medicine), acupuncture (reflexology), homeopathy (home remedies), acupuncture (reflexology), acupressure, homeopathy medicine), acupuncture (homeopathy), acupuncture, homeopathy), acupuncture (reflexology), acupressure, homeopathy), acupuncture, acupressure, acupuncture), acupressure, homeopathy and magnetic therapy. There are many other natural healing options, but these are the best.

Okay. You might want to know what each one of the above items mean. Acupressure is also known as reflexology, which requires pressures to be applied in specific areas of the body. Acupressure refers only to body points; reflexology is about the hands and feet. Each location is related to another part of your body.

For instance, if you have stomach discomfort, you can rub your stomach against your foot. The location is about 2 inches below the base of your bigtoe... that's the bottom part of your foot. Apply pressure as often as you can to relieve your stomach pain for a few seconds.

Aromatherapy:

Aromatherapy utilizes the power of aromas. Even though aromatherapy may have some health benefits, even the best doctors aren't able to fully understand its effects on the brain. Vicks vapour rub is something almost everyone has used once in a while to ease nasal congestion. It is a perfect example how scents can change our bodies. Vicks vapor rub may be safe to use. Eucalyptus, however, is a natural way to clear blocked nasal passages. To crush the Eucalyptus leaves, pour boiling water over them. Keep the soothing vapor in your bowl and head by wrapping a towel around it. Within 10 minutes you will feel great.

Acupuncture:

Acupuncture, the science behind putting needles onto your skin, is the science of acupuncture. You can either put needles into your body, or in your ear. It is possible to use acupuncture in your ears to treat certain diseases or deficiencies. Place a small needle in the area of your liver that you want to heal. The liver is then able to stimulate oxygen-rich bloodflow. The body's natural healing power is also stimulated.

Essential Oils:

Oils either release a soothing aroma, such as aromatherapy or relax the body. Lavender Oil and other oils can be used to rub on the sides or temples of your forehead. They also work on your muscular smell receptors and one of your reflex (reflexology), points. This will reduce pressure absorption through the skin. Lavender Oil can also be applied to your skin and neck to soothe if you don't want to sleep at night. If you are unable to fall asleep, it will help you sleep longer and more comfortably. For anyone just starting out in natural healing, essential oils can be a good first step. There are many benefits to essential oils, but it is easy to remember them all.

Home Remedies:

The word itself says it all. The home remedy refers to everything that surrounds a house that can be used for healing. Home remedies include the use of crushed garlic to treat infections. Use crushed garlic to clean up infected cuts and wounds. You can let it continue for as short as 10 minutes. But stop when the infection is gone. How can you tell if your cut is infected? Commonly, after your cut is done, the wound will bleed to thicken. It will then look golden and smooth when dry. As the body heals, the skin should remain red until it is fully healed. Sometimes, infection can be a problem with larger wounds or bruises. The majority of these diseases are not very serious. However, if they aren't addressed promptly, they can prove to be deadly. BUT don't worry. Now you are familiar with garlic. It is difficult to label home remedies because there are so many options.

Homeopathic:

The amazing benefits of homeopathic medicine are endless. You can absorb healing properties from small pills or tablets by dissolving them in your mouth. Belladonna is an excellent homeopathic drug. It's also great to use if you have a fever. It will reduce symptoms and speed up the recovery process. Homeopathy can be learned quickly and is very easy to use. They are like wearing tics. Drop the right dosage and you will have a better experience. Learn about homeopathy medicine. You can find lots of information online or visit a store that sells homeopathic medicine. Find the homeopathic medicine area and start reading the labels. Every label for homeopathic medicine gives you information about the product and how much it should be taken. This makes it simple to choose the right homeopathic medicine for your needs.

Iridology:

If you don't know what your iris looks like, it's the vibrant part of the eye that surrounds your student. By observing your iris, you can determine the current and future states of your body. You can see the relationship between certain parts of the iris and specific organs. Interesting story about Iridology. In the beginning, a boy played with birds and ran a limb of a bird. He noticed the small line that appeared on the iris in the birds' legs when the leg break occurred because he was near the bird. He was Iridology's founder.

Plants for healing:

Plants can have healing properties. It's very easy to use. To make them easy, you can take dried leaves and crush them. Next, pour boiling water over them. The healing properties of the boiling water are extracted. Once the water has cooled, you can drink it or wait. The healing properties of the water make you beautiful. Boldo is good for upset stomachs. For people who tend to consume spicy or fatty food a lot, Boldo tea is an excellent choice. The Dandelion plant is a great way for blood to cleanse and it will likely grow wherever you are. The Dandelion plant's green leaves can be harvested, washed and added to your salad. You can do this every spring for a few week or whenever your body needs cleaner blood.

Crystal healing

Crystals are elements, minerals, and products of our earth. It's no surprise that crystals can aid in healing. Our bodies are capable of healing themselves through absorption. You can use a healing crystal to heal your skin. But healing crystals have other functions. They enable us to heal ourselves.

Magnetic:

Magnets are extremely powerful. Attractions have incredible power. It doesn't take too much time for me to tell you a story about how appropriate magnets work to heal. A friend of mine discovered a mysterious mole below his left brow. He assumed it was cancerous and went to the doctor to get it checked. He didn't have enough money nor the will to go to the hospital so he decided to try mole removal magnettherapy. By applying a negative magnetic force to the mole, he was eventually able to destroy the cancerous cells. He took three months to get the battery out of its socket. He did this all for free, and it was without any surgery. Magnetic therapy is something we all should use.

Yeah... Wow... There are many natural methods of healing. It is important that we all utilize them, especially today. Healthcare costs are high. It can also take more than a week to just make an appointment. If you have a chronic disease, it means you'll be suffering for up to a week before your body can heal. You don't know much about natural healing methods. Knowing a few of the different healing methods available to you, you can start healing even while you wait for your doctor. You will likely be more well by the time your appointment arrives. Learn now to be able to heal tomorrow.

Chapter 3: Mental Health

W

What does good mental state mean? Although mental health can be described at a very basic level as a mental absence, the entire issue of mental illnesses and mental well-being is complicated and difficult to define. This is how we can define mental health. We can refer to what happens when we have mental illness and are not in good health.

Here in the United Kingdom it is predicted that 25% of the population may become mentally ill during their lifetime. Mental illness can strike anyone, regardless of age, gender, or socioeconomic status. You can get it at any moment, with or without warning. What can you do to determine if your mental illness is present?

Mental illness may manifest in many different ways. No two people will experience the same degree of mental illness. One may experience mild symptoms during their daily life, while another person with mental illness might have severe ones. However, some people might have severe disabilities that prevent them from being able to manage their own lives or be integrated into society.

It is crucial to recognize when someone is mentally ill in order to receive the necessary support. However, recognizing signs that are subtle or unclear can make it difficult to find the right person for you. You can be diagnosed with a mental illness if your mood, attitude, and actions change.

One of the most common ways that our lives can be affected is through depression, anxiety and compulsive behaviors, phobias, panic attacks, manic or bipolar depressions, schizophrenia, or dementia. There are variations, sub-groups, as well as different degrees of severity within each term. Mental illness is often not apparent. Friends and families can misunderstand the symptoms and make it difficult to diagnose. Isolation is possible because the individual cannot comprehend what is happening and why it is being behaved in that way.

What is the root cause of poor mental health?

Although no one knows what causes mental illness, there may be a combination of factors such as environmental and biological conditions that could play a role.

It seems that mental illness is more common in certain groups. This may indicate that some circumstances, such as poverty and other miserable living conditions, disability, people from minority ethnicities, long-term or prisoner status, and others, could trigger mental illness. People who are addicted to or dependent on alcohol are more likely than those who do not suffer from mental illness. Also, different types and forms of mental illness seem to be more familiar to both men and women.

It is possible to become ill from psychiatric illnesses due to life changes. It can also be linked to a genetic component. This is because people with a history mental illness in their families are more likely develop it. Research has also shown that certain forms psychiatric disorders can be made worse by low Omega 3 levels.

There are many factors involved that make it difficult to predict who will develop mental illness. All of us may be affected by mental illness at one time or another.

Support No matter what kind of mental illness, support is available. First and foremost, it is crucial to recognize a problem early. This will help you heal. Some people believe that ignoring a psychiatric condition or suffering is a sign or weakness. They also fear stigmatization, failure, lack knowledge, or even negation. Assistance is necessary because mental illness can not be ignored and symptoms can persist for many years. This can cause unnecessary pain and misery.

Your doctor is the first to call. He will examine you and recommend treatment options. Most mental illnesses can be treated with the help and support of friends and family. Even in severe cases, it is possible to reduce the severity and improve your quality of life with proper diagnosis.

Mental Health Stigma

Although mental health awareness and other mental health issues have increased, there is still a lack of knowledge. Attitudes to Mental Illness 2007 was a government survey that found that over half of those surveyed believed people with mental illness should be admitted to a hospital or in a psychiatric facility. The results showed that attitudes toward people with mental illnesses have dropped since 1994.

Surprisingly many people don't know what mental illness is and how it affects them all, regardless of whether or not they have a diagnosis. If you consider that 25% to 25% of the population suffers from mental health issues at any given time, it is quite possible that we will have someone in our lives who does. It is up to us to know what mental illness is, and what we can get help for it.

People with mental disorders often feel lonely, rejected, or afraid to share their thoughts with others. They are more likely to not receive the support they need, and may become more depressed and even worse. People need to know that mental health does NOT have to stop them from enjoying a better quality of living. It is possible to get help and most people with mental issues will regain full control of their lives.

A new mental-health guide: The Royal College of Psychiatrists has published a new guide to mental health. This guide was published in November 2007 and aims to inform the public what mental illness is. It also represents a significant step toward addressing stigmatization associated with mental illness.

The guide is simple to understand and has been recommended by over 60 mental healthcare professionals. The Mind: a User's Guide covers a broad range of mental diseases and includes a section on nature, diagnosis, treatment, and recovery.

It also pointed out that while the prevalence of mental illness in people who live in socially disadvantaged communities is higher than in other parts of the world, the rate at which stigmatization occurs in these areas remains lower than in other countries. This indicates that confronting mental illness is not enough to change attitudes.

Gender differences are also common. Study done in Scotland found that men with mental disorders were more skeptical of women than men and are more likely to avoid having contact with people who have the same mental disorder. Even among those who showed a positive attitude towards mental health issues, many stated that they were reluctant about speaking to someone with a mental disorder. This only indicates that others' mental health perceptions remain in fear.

KPMG and the Chartered Personnel and Development Institute surveyed over 600 employers in a recent survey. It found that doctors fail to do enough to support people with mental illnesses returning to work. This leads to a loss of billions in the business community. As an example, only 3% rated their doctor support as "outstanding".

One possibility is that doctors don't know much more than what drugs and time off work can do for someone suffering from anxiety or depression. Worse still, 52% said that they had never hired someone with a mental illness history that perpetuates stigma. A more positive side note is that more than half the employers who have hired someone with a mental illness question said their experience was good.

Does attitudes change? While governments and organizations have done a lot in trying to shift public perceptions about mental health, is it enough? Until we understand that mental illness doesn't discriminate, everyone can at any time, regardless of age, sex or social background, be in the stigma associated mental disease.

Mental illness isn't discriminatory. It can affect anyone at any age, regardless of gender or social background. However, mental illness is still stigmatized. Although some government initiatives and awareness campaigns have been successful, there is much more work to be done.

As individuals, we must ensure that we understand and are educated about these issues. Only then can stigmatization of mental health become a thing past.

Holistic Healing - Meaning

Holistic healing calls for a holistic approach in order to overcome disequilibriums and to live a more balanced life. Holistic healing can be used in conjunction with alternative medicine, integrative medicine or complementary medicine. However, it is not a necessary focus for your physical health. However, the perception of discomfort is often what leads to holistic healing.

It is important that we pay attention to pain and other discomforts. It is difficult to overlook the obvious when we are physically hurt. It is obvious that we should attempt to ease our pain. Holistic healing cannot be considered an "alternative" for medical treatment. Sometimes, a doctor will be the best person to help you with your illness.

Holistic Healing addresses all aspects of a person's well-being. It does not only address the physical manifestations of disease.

Holistic healing should not be used as a short-term fix. It is a constant discovery process in search of answers.

Holistic healing goes far beyond the link between mind and body. Holistic healing is a lifestyle. The holistic approach to health goes beyond the link between mind-body.

The overall value of wellness and "wholesomeness" was high. All aspects in a person's daily life (physical recovery, mental well-being, happiness, spiritual beliefs, values and psychological well-being) must be considered. The holistic approach allows us to look for tools that will help us attract our desires and reach personal power.

The person who seeks to be whole within himself quickly learns how important to look after others, care about the planet, have compassion for other people and accept the differences that exist among them.

Holistic healing techniques:

1. Acupressure-

Acupressure can be described as an alternative medicine similar to acupuncture. The theory of energy and life is based on the presence of "meridians". In order to clear blockages in these meridians and treat acupuncture point problems, external pressure may be used. You can use pressure with different tools, such as elbows or manually.

Acupressure is a great way to reduce nausea and vomiting, back pain, tension headaches, stomach upset and other symptoms.

2. Acupuncture

This is an alternative form of medicine. It is essential in traditional Chinese medicine (TCM). Thin needles are inserted into the body at points where acupuncture is performed. These same points can also be used to apply pressure or laser light. Acupuncture works well for pain relief and can also be used in many other conditions.

3. Astrology-

Astrology, the study of the relative movement and position of celestial items as a method of divining people and events, is called Astrology.

4. Bach Flower Remedies-

Bach flower remedies can be water-and/or-brand treatments. They involve high levels of floral dilutions. Bach asserts that the expected healing properties of flowers are preserved by the presence dew in their petals.

The statistical probability of only one molecule remaining after dilution means that the remedies can contain the energy and vibrant nature of the flora. The solutions are sometimes called vibration medicines. They rely on a pseudoscientific concept of water memories. These are homeopathic solutions because they are extremely water-dilutive, but don't follow the same homeopathic principles as the principle of the similar thing.

5. Crystal healing-

Crystal healing is an alternative pseudoscientific process that uses rocks or crystals.

The practitioner places crystals on the body, usually in line with the so called chakras. Practitioners place crystals around the body to help build an energy grid, which is supposed to be healing energy.

6. Reiki cure-

Reiki is an alternative treatment. Since its conception in Japan in 1995, Reiki has been adapted to various cultural traditions. It uses a technique called palm healing. This method is said to transmit "positive energy", which practitioners believe facilitates healing.

Reiki is seen as a pseudo-science. It is based on Qi ("chi"), which can be described as a universal life force.

7. Hypnotherapy-

Hypnotherapy can be described as a type or psychotherapy that induces a subconscious transformation in the patient, such as new emotions, ideas and behaviors. It's done under hypnosis.

Unusual behavioral properties and propensities are found in hypnotized individuals, which include increased suggestiveness, response, and other characteristics.

8. Pranic healing

Pranic Healing is a process where prana (love), can help heal the body's suffering by manipulating the energy fields of the person. Pranic healing, he says, is similar to acupuncture. It treats the power body which in turn affects your physical body.

9. Yoga -

Yoga can be practiced as an alternative medicine or as a form of practice. Hatha yoga is an ancient Indian tradition that includes yoga. This is a type or exercise that has low impact, and can often be used to treat ailments. Yoga can also take place in groups. This may include imagery and respiration, meditation, music, and imagery.

Mental Health Insurance

While public awareness campaigns are important in highlighting the issues of mental health and stigmatization, it is not just the public who suffer from them. People living with a mental illness face discrimination daily from banks, employers, businesses, and even their own families.

The truth is that any individual can develop a mental health issue regardless of their age, race, occupation, and social status. One in four Americans will suffer from a mental disorder within the next year, according to statistics. You can have mild cases of anxiety and depression, as well as more severe cases of schizophrenia and bipolar disorder. Outside, however, there are problems.

One of the most devastating aspects of mental illness is the loneliness, isolation, and social exclusion the sufferer can experience. This is due to the indifference of others. If we look at insurance, which most people take as a given, but not if there is a history of a mental illness or if you are currently dealing with a mental health issue, this could be one example.

An important report on discrimination against mentally ill people shows that insurance companies deny coverage and make exceptions to insurance plans, even though the issues were dealt with years ago. This applies to all types and levels of insurance.

This shows that insurance companies as well as others are often unable to comprehend the facts or reality of mental illness and data. A few mental health issues can arise from a specific situation. Once treated, however, the problem will not recur. Most mental illnesses are short-term and people who seek assistance for mental health issues lead normal, full lives. Most importantly, people don't face greater risk simply because they have a mental disorder. The insurance companies determine their insurance premiums using the perceived risk rate. This rate is supposed not to be based solely on medical evidence. This may be the best area.

What are you going to do about it? If there is disability discrimination, the Disability Discrimination Act can be used to bring legal action. Mind claims that this Act only covers a handful of cases, and many will never succeed. Citizens Advice Bureau says that most insurance claims for compensation do not succeed if mental health is involved. This is because so many policies are omitted.

However, it's not all bad. However, most people realize that something is wrong somewhere and people with mental health issues deserve the same rights. For example, the Mental Health America Association conducted a survey in the US and found that Americans feel that those with mental health problems should not be discriminated against by their insurers. About 96% believe that insurance policies should also cover mental illness. The UK government is fully aware of the exclusion and mental health issues and is working hard to improve the laws in order to prevent unfair discrimination.

However, it is important to remember that mental illness can affect anyone, and can be treated. Without the same protections that all other people with mental disorders have, they will be exposed to the insurance problem.

Mental Health Recovery Keys

It can lead to mental disorders that are demoralizing or paralyzing. There are many ways to maintain mental health, and to recognize mental illness. But these four key recovery factors can be summarized in four easy steps. For the restoration of mental well-being, there are four key elements: employment, accommodation (treatment), medication management trauma treatment and the creation of a network of friends.

Housing is essential for everyone, no matter how sick or well you may be. According to statistics, the proportion of homeless persons with untreated mental illness are high. Worse yet, it is difficult for these people to afford basic shelter. They also have limited access to the right medication, so there is a constant downward spiral. Stable housing is perhaps the most crucial factor in customers' recovery.

This is the right time to discuss with both clients and practitioners how they can help to obtain accommodation. It is essential for psychiatrists to focus on finding affordable and government-subsidized consumers ' homes, ideally when they are removed from their immediate environment (such as being prone to relapse or ongoing use of substances, and so on). There are many places in major cities with low-income apartment buildings that can be accessed by these customers. You must understand that security is vital to all aspects of life. Shelter housing is far better than living in the streets for people with mental disorders. If you are eligible for these payments, an address will be required to obtain employment and social security insurance payments. Housing is crucial to mental health recovery.

Employment is vital to independence and self sufficiency, if housing is available. It is crucial to remember that you shouldn't do it too quickly. It's okay to slow down your reentry into the workforce. If you feel ready, take a part time job and change. This is also a good time to return to school. You will be in better shape if technical skills are available.

Microsoft SQL and Java, Microsoft Access as well as C++, C#, C#, and Python are ideal computer programs for mental healthcare professionals interested in enrolling patients in higher educational institutions. These jobs are demanding, high-paying, and can sometimes be done remotely.

Job management is money management. Persons with mental illnesses should be managed by their family members or a therapeutic funds if they are unable to manage their finances. It is a serious problem. Therefore, if a customer of mental healthcare gives up funding control in order to ensure illegal substances are not acquired, the control program should be safe, properly managed and managed.

The second key to mental recovery is treatment and management. While finding the right drug combination can take time and shift the chemical and hormone balance, it is well worth the effort. Many problems arise from mental health patients misusing their prescriptions. Make sure you take the time and find the right combination for your condition. This will stabilize your symptoms and help keep relevant jobs in place so that you can have housing and independence.

It is essential to build a positive, supportive social network in order to recover your mental health. The most common symptoms of severe psychotic break include isolation and loneliness. There are many people who can help you with your mental illness, including family and friends. American Clubhouses offer a way to build a community. Some customers are disappointed that these groups only meet to speak but they will become productive and more employment-oriented. However, you should not be a part of any social networking that can lead to backwardness.

Housing, education rehabilitation, and the growth of a social network are all key factors to mental recovery. Housing creates employment and affordable housing is made possible by the creation of jobs. Employment allows for the provision of sufficient medication that can aid in recovery. Stabilization is a way to help create work and make housing more affordable. This is all possible thanks to the support of the social networks.

Crystal Healing and The Base Chakra

Chakras are located at the base or root of our spines. The energy extends down through the legs to our feet.

The system controls the entire skeletal system, especially the spine and blood. It has four petals.

Surreal glands can be found in the endocrine system. The Chakra Red and Black Crystals of this Chakra contain the Kundalini. The Chakra crystals are either black or red.

The Base Chakra represents strength and vitality. This center is our connection to the Earth and nature. The base chakra serves as a link between our physical body and the Earth.

This includes all natural issues like skin, senses and sensuality as well as violence and self defense. Basic survival instincts: the instinct to hunt and for protection. It is the combination the base chakra and this basic self preservation instinct that give it a value of will to live. The Chakra, where the Spirit and matter meet is described because it covers a lot of our physical existence. For spirit and matter to exist, they must meet. The Etheric bodies contain an energy stream that runs between the lower and higher carcasses. The lower pads are found below the diaphragm. The higher pads are higher. Each Chakra lower has its corresponding higher Chakra. The higher Chakras allow for energy transfer from lower Chakras to higher Chakras. The Chakra moved power from a chakra of crown to a Chakra. When the charges have been balanced, the colors will be vivid.

Disorders that are related to Base Chakra an unbalanced include Anorexia-Bulimia- Base-Depression- Cold Hands and Feet-Constipation-Crohn's Kidney Stones-Obesity- High Blood Pressure-Sciatica-Varicose Veins the Base Chakra is connected to protection and the sense of willpower to touch. Your crystals can be used in conjunction with exercise, yoga and massage. These effects will help balance your Chakras.

Specific issues can cause the Base Chakra to become imbalanced. If your Base Chakra imbalance is severe, you may feel disorganized and unspoken or feel disconnected.

The following list shows how healthy your Base Chakra really is. Any column in the positive column means your Base Chakra is healthy. It will also indicate that your Base Chakra could be out-of-control.

POSITIVES

The Base Chakra should be one of your first chakras. It is responsible for bringing harmony.

NEGATIVES: aggression-self-pity-egotistical, Sadistic, domineering-greedy. It is possible to heal your Chakra completely.

Points to Mental Health Care Reform

The critical moment in reforming health care is now when people are more aware of the number of people who have psychiatric problems and those with alcohol problems. They know the importance to address the health care needs of people with severe mental disorders and fulfill the behavioral health needs for all Americans. This helps to create a happier mental health community, and also sets the stage for precedent-setting challenges for mental health agencies across the United States. they are committed in providing support for Member Organizations and states, as well federal agencies and consumer groups, to ensure that people with mental and substance problems face critical challenges.

Many mental agencies at both the community and national level have been meeting regularly to discuss and read about equality and mental healthcare reform legislation. Their work continues and their results are a guide for the lobbying organizations for healthcare reforms.

MENTAL SERVICE

1. Capacity building

2. Personal health centers will need to be integrated into primary health practices.

3. Peer Advisors and Customer Operated Services. Peer Advisors and Customer Operated Services are expected to grow. They will also

include individuals in mental health and drug abuse treatment.

4. With the support of the Patient-Centered Outcomes Research Institute (PCORI), as well as other research initiatives and implementation efforts, it will increase the speed of mental and drug use promotion. This involves, for example, encouraging people with mental illnesses to find a nearby mental health clinic.

MENTAL HEAT MANAGEMENT PROGRAM

5. Medicaid expansion, health exchanges: States need to make major changes to increase the value and quality of drug and mental health programs as their Medicaid networks evolve for expansion. The Exchanges for new Medicaid models, agreements, or billing services must be available to program agencies.

6. Sponsored Employer plans for health and equal chances: Benefits managers, employers, and employees will have to redefine the use behavioral healthcare services in order to combat absenteism. Firms will need adapt their services in order to meet the needs of their

customers and to work closely with their billing and contracting process.

7. Re-design. Payers will support and sometimes even require the creation and implementation of new management structures in order to support healthcare reforms. These include accounting agencies, redesign of the health plan, and guidelines for mental health and substance misuse. ACOs in communities should be owned by provider organizations.

INFRASTRUCTUREMENTALHEALTHCARE

8. Promotion of quality in mental health: Organisations such as National Quality Forum have accelerated the development and implementation of a national quality plan that combines both mental and drug intake measures. This is intended to increase the availability of mental services, reduce costs, and improve community safety and control. Infrastructure will be required by the providers.

9. Information Technology on Health. Both federal and state HIT initiatives need to reflect the importance and impact of mental and

substance use services. These should include providers of mental and drug services, as they will need to provide data for infrastructure design, funding, and design. They will be required to link electronic records and patient identifications to local health data networks, and exchanges of relevant health information.

10. Healthcare Payments Reform - Payers and plans must create and implement new payment mechanisms, including cash, capitation, and that include value-based purchases and value-based design strategies to support mental health and drug abuse. Companies will need to modify their processes, payment systems and work procedures in order comply with these new frameworks.

11. Workforce development: This will include major efforts to address issues such as drug use and mental health, including the expansion of peer advisers. The Workforce Advisory Committee's work will also be considered. Provider organizations must invest and be prepared to grow their workforce in order to meet emerging demand.

Chapter 4: Crystal Therapy: Updated

W

Crystal Healing Works Crystal therapy and treatment have been studied so thoroughly that the scientific community thinks it is deceitful. Millions of people have tried it, and they are happy with the results.

This is why there is such a disparity. The reason crystal therapy doesn't work is because it relies on pseudo-scientific claims. It can have a significant effect in other environments. This was thought to be a placebo effect.

It's not impossible to say that something was created by the placebo effect or psychosomatic. Psychology is real science. Real science. Actual conditions such as anxiety or stigma can have real physical and emotional effects. It does not render crystal therapy less useful or more effective in the care of patients.

Which Crystals?

Humans love shiny things. We are sensitive to light refraction and colors. Only cats and birds react to crystal light. Refractions are fascinating because light is healthy for us.

They also love water to multiply their species. Different crystals store, channel, and behave differently.

Also, we know that an object attached to a target/object is an excellent tool to focus and envision.

You get many benefits from crystals such as light playing, color, heat channelsing, and a focus tool. This is how we get superhuman abilities.

Let's just be clear, magic properties. The assumptions that scientists have made about almost everything are based on the assumption of a world without an intelligent, capable Supreme Being (SWT). This is great as it eliminates the need to recite mystic nonsense when things are not clear. God(SWT), cannot tell you something. Experimentation and observation are the only way to determine exactly what happens.

Although this is a great thing in many sciences, it is not as sweet in psychology, or any other area that is driven by one's mind or heart. Many people in the world believe some form of belief system. Many atheists believe religion is valid but not based on any physical evidence.

Because no one has been able proof or disprove God's existence, it is up to us to choose whether we want to be atheists and totally abandon all behavior that is based in God's existence (SWT) or what works for us as individuals who believe or at the very least believe that God exists.

If we believe that there are many honored traditions in healing or therapy, then we should not discount them. It is crucial to analyze the motivations.

Zweiten, any scientific argument that is misleading, misinformed or just plain false should be thrown out of our profession. Pseudoscience and psychology Crystals don't produce any more energy that other stones. Their exposure to energy made them crystals, not just gems. Everything that we associate with ordinary rocks can be extraordinary by itself. Crystals are just as attractive to us.

An updated crystal therapist should also be a qualified mineral therapist. We must examine how the beautiful crystals and many types of minerals can impact different people's moods, physical, and mental well-being. It can be helpful for some to have a solid foundation and focus on their goals using a piece of hardened, raw granite.

Some people enjoy sand playing more than others. It is well-known that gardens of rock and sand can be very therapeutic. Burial practices and the sandbox with a glittering diamond can help someone solve difficult problems.

If someone is struggling with trust and body image, it might help to let go of those issues and love yourself as you are. Feel raw diamonds (please do not buy conflict diamonds) on your skin. Even at the commercial level, diamonds are stunning. They might not be the most desirable to show but they still shine and are just as enjoyable. It communicates a positive message.

Undiscovered benefits Crystals can conduct soul energy and have untapped benefits. You can use us to stay focused on one goal and filter out unconscious knowledge from the conscious mind. We also give strength to others.

This assumption is actually based in theology. Science isn't. It doesn't have to.

But faith pure? However, it isn't pure faith. It is supported by physical evidence. Make use of crystal and other mineral treatments. But, the only way to make it work is with crystals and rocks. In each case, the crystals provided guidance, focus and increased the positive energy of the situation.

The field is generally accessible. Just go out and do the work. If you are open-minded, your practice will be much more successful and fulfilling.

Methods and Techniques of Medical Astrology

Medical astrology refers to the branch of astrology that deals specifically with the client's health and disease potential. People frequently consult an astrologer in times when life is going through significant changes.

When do I get to be part of my heritage?

Do I have to ask him/her for a marriage? Etc. A lot of people visit the medical Astrologer when they are in the advanced phases of their disease. Often, this is after some surgery and after a long history of dealings with physicians. The usual questions that the medical specialist will ask you are: Should surgery be performed?

Does it have to be an operation

When should this procedure be done?

Why don't people have children?

What is the best way to get rid of cancer?

Is there a chance that my cancer will be discovered this year? Etc. You can also predict the course and duration of a particular disease by matching astrological events and arrangements. We can then classify the astrological reason for the disease and determine the therapy needed. It is often the reverse: clients attend the usual astrology sessions, but before the disease manifests, the astrologer considers the client's horoscope a danger.

A variety of standards are attached to the medical astrologer's advice. No matter if an operation is performed, whether chemotherapy is done or not, radiology is used or not...

"I have a Tuesday appointment for radiation therapy. Should I attend?" "The doctor recommended that I have my bladder removed to stop the spread and spread of cancer. Should this be done? If you cannot deal with serious terminal diseases, and you don't wish to have to live with the consequences of your choice, don't do it. If you're not a professional medical doctor, you need to prepare. You will need to read and research the literature, find information on the Internet, consult with medical professionals, join forums, and participate in membership sites. In an ideal universe, astrologers recommend that customers change their behavior in order to use the extra energy they provide the planets or stars. Some medical astrologers can be more accurate, specific, and smelly, which could indicate that particular crystals, herbs, or remedies are available. It is best not mix the professional astrologers with physicians. If the astrologer and the client are not medical doctors or homeopaths, then the client is not the one to heal. The medical astrologer should never be considered a physician.

The medical astrologer can use all astrological techniques and methods to deduce the nature of an illness. He/she should be a professional astrologer and order. They should also use a broad range of astrological techniques for the benefit of the consumer. The astrologer should not only give advice on healing but also know the natal charts of their clients. In an ideal world, he/she should be connected with healers and doctors to determine which person should be seen next. However, it is preferable that the customer chooses their own doctors and curators after a visit to the astrologer. This way, if something does not go according to plan, the astrologer will be accused as working with the patient's health care provider.

You can agree on which therapy to use from the charts. Signs Signs represent the 12 major systems in the human body. Signs can include the planets. These signs may be detected either at birth or via advanced Horoscopes. There is a salt tissue for each mark. These salt tissues are the building blocks of the human body, organs, and the materials that allow for the creation of tissues, organs, and the whole body. The combination of these salts in material or homeopathic dosages can significantly improve one's health.

A particular food type is the best for each mark. Astrologers who are trained in nutrition can advise consumers on how to improve their health. Doctrine theory, which is the finding of similarities between body and zodiac signs, allows signs to link to herbs that can be prescribed to the patient.

Medical Astrology Horoscope Decades Each sign has thirty degrees. Each degree links to one area of the body by a 360-degree connection.

The world within this degree is more susceptible to disease. The degree will tell us which part of your body is infected while the planet will indicate which type of condition. You can link degrees and midpoints.

Each individual planet is a source of energy in the horoscope. Mars has a firelike quality, so it lights up the body's fires (which results in high temperature) and purifies it. Pluto stands to represent unknown bacteria. Neptune, however, stands for medically-recognized bacteria. The behavior of the asteroids, especially those larger than Juno Ceres, is similar. The Uranian planets are also useful in medical astrology. There are 8 Uranian "Uranian", which have no astronomical data and whose influence is strong in the chart. These planets can have clear medical connotations which may increase the accuracy of scientific astrology studies by up to 90%.

Five of the 12 houses used in daily astrology have greater significance than the other. They are the first house-the human body, the sixth house illnesses, and the eighth house-support.

The ninth house is for people with terminal conditions. The twelfth house is for isolation. It can also be associated with psychic problems, hospitals, monasteries, and autoimmunity.

Medical astrology has a special meaning for every home.

1-- consciousness, face brain tumors brain insults, and/or consciousness

2-- Blood, eating habits, electrolytes. Hormones, pituitary disease and diabetes.

3-- Speech problems, the lungs

4-- food production. Mom, milk. Biology. Ancestry.

5-- Heart, myocardial and/or heart attack.

6--Cancer, daily living, personal hygiene, and nutrition

7-- brain problems death, body balance, spine,

8-- Removing processed foods, adrenaline cortex. pituitary and kidney.

9-- the upper half of the brain

The house ruler is the main indicator of house-related happenings, while the planets of the house are less relevant. For example, consider the sixth and its ruler. Its position, its aspects and its transits are all important to understand what types of diseases could be. Only after the dictator has been placed under significant strain can we begin predicting the presence of a particular disease.

Aspects of planetary life How a planet transmits its energy depends primarily upon its relationships with other planets. These planets must be at the same angle as the two in the middle of the circle. A combination Sun/Saturn will slow down metabolism while Mars and Sun make it easy to consume their energy. People who are involved in sport often have a slower metabolism.

Moon degrees are particularly harmful. Two planets linked together can lead to various health problems. Malefic planets and the Sun have the most cancerous elements. The malefic quadrants and Saturn squaring Saturn on the Moon give cancer predisposition. However, malefic aspects from Neptune to Pluto on the Moon might also cause the same effect. Malignancy is a form of cancer, as it is in other branches. It's always useful to look at the functional aspects as they can provide changes and often a full cure. This is often done through treatments or people like the explanation (e.g. trine of Neptune-healing by an apothecary). If the rulers and representatives of the sixth, eighth, and twelveth houses are not making a difference, then we need to find the right people. If he is a doctor, he will heal.

Medical Astrology Midpoints A planet lies at the midpoint of two distant worlds. There is a unique medical line for each midpoint: Saturn and Jupiter mean the liver, Saturn and March mean spasms, death and more. Midpoints are essential to making every chart unique. Without them, medical astrology will be difficult. In order to achieve greater precision in the following charts, you should include the Uranian Planets and their Centers.

Scientific aphorisms. The Medical Aphorisms are general settings for certain diseases and conditions. As an example, Mars near the Ascendant in Scorpio (or any squared malefic in Gemini or Saturn) is going be predisposed to bronchitis. Medical astrologers must be able to identify such combinations in the chart. However, they won't be able to bear the sight of the manual at the end of a session.

The astrology application on the natal maps can now calculate medical conditions. It would be more difficult to do medical-astrology without this piece of software. There are hundreds of them.

Natal Chart Diagnosis of an Illness Each chart has dozens configurations that may prove difficult to interpret. It doesn't mean that a person should be considered sick simply because they have all of the diseases in the diagram. If at least three inclinations simultaneously are active, the configuration will cause illness. A square between Saturn or the Moon can lead to cancer. Because it takes seven long years for the advanced Moon's malignant features to manifest in the natal Saturn, the second predisposition might be every seven. The solar chart, which can show a relation between Saturn and the Moon, can provide the third variable. Another option is a slow transit by Saturn, which could bring the third factor to fruition. If all four of these variables are present at the same moment, the consumer may feel that he is in an evil circle and can't find his way home.

If we see a concentration of about similar transits, we are unable to alert the customer about cancer or other severe diseases. We can measure solar charts and transits ahead of time so we can tell the client exactly when problems are starting and ending.

Sometimes, similar predispositions can occur from different configurations. A combination of surgery may be required when Uranus is square to the Ascending and Pluto also has the Ascending Square. Now, it is enough for Mars transit to make one of them or Mars appear in the solar returning chart at the Uranus/Plutu midpoint. It seems that surgery cannot be avoided.

Transit, Growth, Salary, and Synastry Diagnosis in native Astrology. We use only the native charts and the transits in 90% our workshops. There is simply not enough time to look into all the useful charts in one-on-1 sessions. Medical astrology can use multiple maps. The diagram does not matter if there are three separate confirmations of disease. If you are looking for clues in a graph, it can be a tedious task before you discover the star that caused the symptoms. If you connect facts in real life to their astrological origins you can predict how the disease will unfold.

Long transits from malignant planets can cause all manners of health issues. A positive horoscope is the best way to see the long-term future of a customer. Because of strong accents, which can last only a few days but can often continue throughout the client's lives, medical astrology uses solar charts.

It's important to choose the right people to stay with. Customers share their energy with those they care about. Sometimes they are able to cure customers by being present. Sometimes, they can make the customer even sicker. Also, the horoscopes of each country can be consulted.

Auxiliary Astrology Techniques Arabic Parts are created by adding two points to which one is subtracted and subtracting the third. There are approximately 500 Arab components, some of which are directly related to the health. Pars Fortunae, which combines Sun-Moon and Ascendant influences, is the most prominent Arab part.

Every house has its Arabic collection. The sixth house contains two Arabic pieces that are of medical and astrological interest.

Hourly Astrology can produce a lot information. The diagram is constructed using horary Astrology. It uses natal diagrams, and the derived diagrams. It is not possible to read a plan diagram without first reading the natal pictures and all the other tables. It's worth spending some time learning astrology. This can give you an insight into the actual situation, how the disease is progressing, any possible surgeries and death, and so on. If we know the time when the infection occurred, then this is possible. It also has its own rules.

Electional Astrology attempts to predict when the action will begin. Diagrams can be used to analyze medical astrology charts and determine when the prescribed treatment should start.

Modern medicine has medical astrology as a role. They can calculate the patient's situation at the time and then predict whether it will be good or bad. It doesn't deal with the patient's future, and it is almost always used when something horrible has occurred. Astrology Medical is the missing piece between the patient's diagnosed diagnosis, the current treatment, as well as the future direction of the disease. The astrological prognosis is available in advance. This means that something can also be done ahead of time. Homeopathy and other energy-healing systems are the natural continuation of medical astrology. They "spend" the unwanted but current energy that the stars or planets are sending to us through the astral corpe. Medical of astrology's greatest advantage is its ability to not only predict which remedies or techniques may be effective, but also to stop them and make use of specific healing methods.

Clearing Crystals For Crystal Healing

Crystal healing can be described as a healing method that involves crystals being placed on or all around the receptor's skin. This treatment technique is used to treat and restore strength to the body since ancient times. These crystals are good for energy healing and help to release negative energy.

Ayurveda records in India from Ancient Egypt provide the first evidence of this method of healing. It has been used in China for approximately 5000 years.

Crystals are described to be the gift of nature to humanity, and they promote healing. They are available in every color, size, and combination. You can see that every crystal has an amazing vibrational resonance. Each crystal is unique. They all have unique mineral contents, colors, and intrinsic geometry that contribute to their uniqueness.

The relation. The vibrational energy system of the human body, also called a dynamic electricity system, is part of the relationship. Crystals and the Human Body Thanks to nature crystals are excellent electromagnetic conductors that can interact very well in humans' electromagnetic systems. It is believed that crystals transmit vibrations to activate various energy centers in the human body's electromagnetic system. These vibrations can have a positive effect on the entire system.

Crystal Healing-Crystal Cleaning but sometimes, a crystal once attracted another doesn't seem so. Crystals that are not attracted to someone may need to be cleaned. Clearing a stone or crystal is necessary before it can release or emit all its power. A crystal that is cleared emits positive emotions while a clogged crystal is tingly-cold. Sometimes, a blocked or removed crystal can feel hot or heavy.

Crystal healing involves purifying stones and crystals by a number of means.

Moonlight-An effective method to remove crystals. Bring them in the full moon outside. To dissipate this energy, we suggest decreasing moons. But you can do it any time. The time taken depends on the healing practitioner's tolerance as well as the size and shape of the rock or crystal. It's a great idea to place a ring on a tree during the moonlight.

Another way is to bury the crystal deep in the earth, especially if it is very dirty or you want to blow the glass. A qualified healer must approve crystals or gemstones in order to make crystal healing work.

Crystal Healing's effectiveness in Balancing Mind & Bodily

Crystal cure is not a replacement for time-honored medication, particularly when it comes to sudden unplanned crises that have repeated themselves over and over. It will undoubtedly help you settle into the ambulance and get to the hospital. Our bodies contain a powerful yet not fully realized self healing technique. The healing power of crystals is a way to activate your natural healing abilities. There are no harmful side effects. You cannot even pay the price for a diamond. You will find yourself interested in the healing and maintenance of crystals. Don't stop your enthusiasm and get going.

Crystals can be used for healing and to increase the healing potentialities. These gorgeous stones can be used by themselves or together with Reiki's treatment form or any other type of medical assistance. They can be found around the world. They can be found in many different forms of quartz, from jade (a valuable gemstone that requires high-polishing) to rubies ("deep and brilliant red gems") Clear quartz crystal, which is the most popular stone used to heal and calm, can also be used for other purposes.

When talking about crystals' working mechanisms, these valuable stones can be used for cleansing, balancing, or reinforcing all healing energies. Each crystal has its own characteristics and vigor. One example is precise quartz. This crystal balances and syncs your body and creates negative energy in your network. Hematite can be used to stabilize your body and avoid negativism. These energies, which are crystals in nature, can be reacted with your strength.

The healing properties of crystals can be applied to your body in many ways. If you are ill, you can use crystals to heal yourself. Reiki crystal healing can be used to relax the whole body. Reiki practitioners used crystals to place on the chakras (centers that hold spiritual power) of the body to expend negative energy and restore divine and earthly energies. A number of religious and massage healers use crystals. You can learn how to use them.

Crystal healing is a form or replacement for health care. Your doctor's advice is important. Learn about alternative herbal remedies, such as crystal therapy, and then incorporate them into your own life. Your mind and body can be rejuvenated in a natural way. Spend your time learning about crystal healing and incorporating it into your life. Use crystals is a personal decision. Do not force others to use them.

The Art Of Crystal Healing and Reiki

The practice of crystal healing was based heavily on subtle energy. The body's electromagnetic or bio magnetic field surrounds it is known as subtle energy.

Sometimes Reiki practitioners can use crystals. Many stones are placed on different parts of your body, including the abdomen and front. The stones were designed to dissolve mental, cognitive, religious and spiritual barriers that prevent well-being.

The practitioner's job is to be compassionate and non-judicatory to the client. To give you the safety to express your emotions and to protect you from harm, This is considered part and parcel of the healing process. The energy released by the crystals is something you should be paying attention to after you place them on your body during a Reiki session. You can see that the body has an aura or its own unique energy. Crystals such as rubies and diamonds are also a part of this energy. Be aware that every form of stone will be unique and have minor variations.

There have been crystal healing teachings for millennia. Ancient cultures like the Egyptians, Chinese, and Indians believe in the power crystals can bring. They believed that certain stones could be used to heal, protect and enhance their sense of awareness.

Many crystals can have their combined energy. They will most likely absorb people's power or the surrounding environment. If your crystal is carrying negative energy, you will want to purify it to remove the harmful energies.

Here are three easy ways you can wash your crystals.

* Sunlight: Put your crystals out in the sunlight to shine. Tip: Because of the possibility of amethyst stones fading in sunlight, do not place them in the sun.

* Water filtered

* Salt: Cover the salt crystals with salt. Throw away the salt after it's finished.

Even though it's important to clean out your crystals regularly, you may need to charge them occasionally. The way it works is that charging a Crystal means giving it power. To bring power to your crystal, the following strategy is possible: hold the crystal in one hand, send Reiki with the symbol Cho Ku Rei (e.g., Cho Ku Rei) at least three times, either softly or loudly. Cho Ku Rei is a Japanese word that can be used to calm down.

Crystal healing therapy could be a good option if you want to relax your body and mind.

Chapter 5: Healing Gemstones & Crystals: Inspiring Well-Being And Balance

O

The mystical and curative powers of crystals have been used by holistic healers for many years. It does not matter if it is to restore harmony or well-being in your life or for your clients. The healing power of gemstones is not limited to holistic healers. People are beginning to recognize the value of gems and begin to use them in their lives. But, how can you identify the best crystals and gemstones to suit your needs?

It can be difficult to find the perfect gems for you. But once you learn about their history and strengths, it is possible to select the best pearls. Since ancient times, the primary use of gems and crystals was for healing or spiritual reasons. Jewels were not common in those days. The jewels were only made available to a small number of people. They are available to everyone who requires them, which is a good thing.

Many people are skeptical of the healing powers of gems. Modern science acknowledges the impact of gemstones, and crystals. These crystals are found in lasers, watches and computers as well as in water. This support for science is not enough to determine their ability to support healing of the body.

The magnetic strength of crystals and gems varies. Many of them have incredible healing properties that can be used for human form therapy. It is well known that these gems emit tiny vibrations and frequencies which have the potential to profoundly affect our lives. Gems are used in many religions to harmonize, balance, heal, and transform the mind and heart. It is used in many ways that can help us relax, improve, and stabilize ourselves.

However, because of the incredible healing properties of gemstones, many people still use them for their healing. How to purify gems from past energies is one of the most important things you need to know about them.

Leave the gem for six to eight hour under running water. You can also put them in a hole in the earth and leave them there overnight. Otherwise, you can put them on a lamp's flame to melt. For purification, your gemstone should be placed in direct sunlight once it has been cleaned. This is because it is an exceptional power source.

Remember to wear your rock. If you store your stones in a jewelry box, they won't be much use. You will be able to heal your mind and soul with the help of a healing stone that you keep with you all the time. The only thing that is required is to keep the stone in your hands and allow it to work.

If you are looking for information about therapeutic gemstones you need to be open-minded. Although there are many theories as to how gems work (and some of them can be confusing and overwhelming), there are still many options. Be a believer in the stones. Let the energy work as it should.

Information about a new stone is important for everyone, no matter how old you are. You have the option to choose from many gemstones or crystals. Many of the most famous stones and their techniques are not well-known.

* Rose Quartz is most common healing gemstones. It's well-known for its gentle healing energies. This gemstone is mostly used to heal your heart. It's used to protect your heart from pain, emotional heartbreak therapy, and other types of heart problems. It is also a blessing for people who are trying to love their own selves.

* Fluorite, another common stone in the group of gemstones. It comes in many colors and can be used to protect people from adverse effects. It can absorb any negative energies in the area and help keep them at a distance. It is recommended that you wash your stones at least once a week, especially stones that have been deemed to remove negative energies.

* Lapis: A top dog in gemstone world. It's believed to release mysteries and can be used to help users with emotional blocks and confusion.

* Hematite - A mineral many people use. It is the unmistakable metallic silver-gray color for all gemstones. It is often used to ground those who wish escape from all the troubles and activities of this world by taking flight.

* Amethyst, a lovely purple stone, is often linked to spiritual healing. It is believed to improve the awareness and knowledge of its clients.

* Jade is used to encourage acceptance and calm the mind. It helps to motivate individuals to place less importance on themselves and others.

* Turkish: This is a stone that can be used only to create jewelry elegance. It can be used as a teaching rock. It is an often used stone for meditation and dream experiences.

* Cyanate can be used by professional gemstone-healer professionals. It is best to wear it near the chakras of the chest. It is used for channeling and opening contact centers. This beautiful gemstone can, and will, purify its

self of negative energies like many other gemstones.

* Citrine, another top-ranked gemstone. It is a beautiful yellow stone that can help you achieve your goals. It is believed to help you attract wealth and personal energy.

* Obsidian can be used again as a protective or grounding agent. It is believed that it can bring about change and serenity.

* Amazonite: This gemstone is used to increase self-value.

* Amber is used to reduce stress and anxiety. It will help you experience joy again.

* Apatite, another stone used to promote communication within your world. It is used in situations where a misunderstanding has occurred and can help to calm any tension that results from a struggle.

* Green Aventurine: Used for physical treatment. It's used over the most distressing parts of the body.

* Blue Aventurine - This is used to improve blood circulation.

* Coral is used to express feelings.

* Diamond: Not just for women! It's used for personal clarity.

* Emerald is used for healing, both mentally and physically. It is one the most powerful healing gems.

* Carnelian - Used to enhance imagination and cognitive cycles

* Grey Moonstone is used to concentrate rocks, which allows them to have the power and strength of the moonstone.

* Moss Agate - Used to touch the nature and as a foundation stone in meditation.

* Mexican Onyx, which is used for insomnia and support of sleeping conditions.

* Black opal is a rock that helps to concentrate the soul and mind.

* Ruby is also associated with romance and love. It acts as the heart chakra for making love feel.

* Sapphire: A lovely stone known for clarifying minds.

Buy a healing stone to remind you about the healing power of gemstones. They will assist you in understanding healing gemstones. The experience you might have had is an important step in using your healing power.

Crystals and Wicca

Following Wicca tradition, crystal divine moon gemstones have different magical and therapeutic powers. This is an ideal field for solo practitioners, who can freely work with the most potent gemstone and crystal correspondences.

As with plants it is nearly impossible to compile all the crystals and all their definitions. These are however some of the most popular.

Agate-Achates, which is connected to the earth aspect, has healing powers that can help with depression and energy. Magical associations allow agate to generate truth and new insights. This helps overcome sadness, loneliness, and other negative emotions.

Amber can be combined with the element of Fire and the Sun to treat eye- and throat problems. It gives clarity, trust protection, strength, and security.

Amethyst: Associated with the water dimensions, amethysts provide astrological connections for Aquarius and Pisces sign a born under. It is used for treating stress, anxiety and depression.

Bloodstone-Bloodstone (also known as heliotropes) is linked to all blood and circulatory system issues associated with the factor of fire. It is a healing stone and can magically work to improve fertility, abundance and wealth.

Carnelian-An object of grounding. Carnelian is believed to have a healing effect on infertility, impotence, and excessive bleeding. It protects the bearer from any supernatural attack by acting as a shield.

In conjunction with the elements Air/Fire, diamond-diamonds have healing powers that can be used to treat sexual dysfunction and reproduction. It is used for intuitive work, meditation, screaming, and astral travel.

Garnet-Fire, genetics the rock most closely associated with Persephone Goddesses. It is often used to treat fertility problems.

Hepatitis -- Hepatitis is a protective, especially from home stone. It's associated with fire and can be used to treat infections, inflammation, fever, and blood disorders. It gives users trust and motivates them to solve problems.

Jade Jade is also used to encourage immortality.

Jasper Jasper is associated to the Earth. It can be used for blood disorders and cancer therapies. It can also serve as a grounding and ritualistic stone. This stone is good luck for the person who carries it.

Lapis Lazuli, a stone linked to the water part, lapisisis used to raise spirits and cure depression. By using magic practices, such as meditation and/or trance work lapis transforms your mind and binds you to the divine.

Moonstone-A waterstone that is closely associated with Moon, this stone has many curative qualities for women. It is used to perform rituals of the Goddess, especially those of wisdom or intuition.

Obsidian - Obsidian, a stone of Fire, can be used to eliminate toxins from your body, particularly the liver. It's a powerful stone for magic and intuition.

Opal-Opals can be replaced by any crystal. They are used for healing all elements and in spiritual and emotional healing. They are protective stones that enhance magic function and absorb energy from all sources, both positive and negative.

Quartz, Rose Rose Quartz, and Quartz are air stones of the heart. They can help you heal your love and relationship problems. His magical powers include everything, from romance to friendship.

White Quartz, Quartz -- White quartz can be used as a medium to connect with the Divine during healing rituals. It is a pillar that promotes intuition, spiritual development, and growth. Sapphires-Always associated with water and used as a treatment for throat and respiratory problems, sapphires are magically used in communication and prophetry with spirit guides.

Tiger's Element Stone Fire (Tiger's Eye) is an element that enhances the physical health of the animal. It's magically used in brave and defensive rituals.

Turquoise-a water-related rocks, turquoise can treat stomach and eye issues, as well as heal broken bones. It can be used to heal, gain wisdom, and develop divine intuition.

Zirconium zircones are used in holistic healing, as well as rituals of love, beauty and harmony. Due to their close resemblance to diamonds, zircons may be used as replacements for certain traditional traditions.

There is no set way to find a stone that suits your needs. Individuals have to decide what stones they want. The best way to deal with rocks is to use their intuition and treat them quickly.

Set a rock/stone under running water. Let it stay out in the sunlight at night. Cover it with salt or let it rest in the Sun for several hours.

Myriad Colors of Crystals, and Their Healing Properties

It is possible to safely say that crystals are as numerous as colors, even though this fact is not known. Each type of crystal has its own healing story, and this is similar to Chinese medicine shops who specialize in herbal blends for all types of ailments.

What crystal do you need to select for a particular purpose? Below is a list of many of the crystal systems that are most used for their application: amethyst-(purple/violet)-This crystal stimulates the immune and endocrine system. It helps to alleviate mental disorders and anxiety and improves the psychological and channeling ability. The amethyst stone is extremely relaxing and is considered a relaxation stone.

Aventurine - Aventurine is purifying. It helps with anxiety and fear relief and promotes autonomy.

Carnelian-(bright yellow)-This stunning vivid crystal enhances nostalgia and soothes sorrow. It boosts imagination, courage, and reduces fear, envy, rage, and anger. Carnelian Crystal is carried by most people for their safety and good fortune. It's a great way to find your right friend.

Fluorite-(milky, light, or slate gray) - Fluorite crystal properties provide protection for your teeth and bones. These are "natural" crystals, which also protect the blood vessels and spleen from toxic substances. Fluorite is also known to "fling back" and produce excessive energy. They are suitable for concentration, mental development, and meditation. Fluorite will keep you healthy and safe when communicating with interdimensional entities, especially if you are involved in interplanetary communication.

Clear Quartz-(white and transparent)- Clear Quartz crystal might be the most widely used because of its simplicity. This remarkable crystal activates and boosts the pineal-pituitary glands which regulate growth. It is highly recommended for children and teenagers. These crystals are also a powerful emotional "balance", enhancing vision and improving thinking. You can place these crystals into a window for all energy levels to activate, especially when you feel-these diamonds have advantages for the disseminating of negative energy.

Lapis-(topaz/blue)-As this crystal is also called, Lapis Lazuli is beneficial for internal organisms: use it if you have a headache, acid reflux, or other gastrointestinal diseases or if you suffer from bloating. It's also beneficial for spiritual development.

Hematite - (Silver/Dark grey)-Hematite is very beneficial for bloodstream smoothflow. It eliminates toxins, stimulates the spleen activity and regulates red blood cells. Hematite is used to ease stress and strengthen the physique.

Rose quartz-(rose/pink)-This crystal is often found near the bed since fertility is believed to increase, and sexual and emotional imbalances are alleviated. It can eliminate anger, frustrations fear, remorse, fear and envy. You have a hot temper? Or a friend who gets too hot? Take a crystal of Rose quartz! Its ideal description is "Everything Sweet," because it promotes forgiveness, love, compassion, and kindness. It's not there without it.

Jasper-(light-brown)-The Jasper crystal is said to be a powerful emotional and psychological healer and promotes harmony and peace. Some believe that it can reveal hidden desires, hopes, or fears. It can improve artistic imagination, so hold it in your hand as you meditate.

It is associated to love and protection. Moonstone-(cream / often bluish-green).

Obsidian-(black/gray)-This brilliant crystal is standard for the sake of calmness and purity for people who either hold, wear, or use it for healing purposes. It is a positive and a negative emotion that can be felt in times of change or transition.

Sodalite - (blue/clear or dark blue) - This beautiful crystal acts as an internal healing agent, affecting the pancreas. It is also believed to help with fear reduction and the ability to balance the male/female polarities or Yin / Yang polarities.

Tiger Eye-(brown/striped/tan/yellow)-This is another crystal that many people use to improve their health: tiger-eye crystals are almost complete: spleen, pancreas, intestines, and colon. It's focused and centering. Are you looking for a stubborn friend to help you? One of these can be placed in the friend's bag. Soon they'll be able see clearly and will feel a sense of perspective.

The Significance Of Crystals In Reiki Courses

Reiki practice uses CrystCitrine. However, crystals are an essential part of the Reiki experience. Reiki is based around changes in energy fields and can be enhanced by matching Reiki crystals. The crystals are pretty, but their primary purpose is to heal Reiki.

There are many crystals you can use in Reiki.

Amethyst is a lovely purple-colored to light-colored gem that resonates strongly with Reiki. Aventurine aids in raising the consciousness of God. Blue Lace Agate is a stone that can both heal and nurture. Reiki courses show that the rock has been used in soothing for many years.

Citrine is another Reiki crystal. It has a pale yellow to orange hue. Reiki courses teach you that Citrine leads towards knowledge and strength.

Clear quartz. Reiki courses suggest that you wash and remove stones.

Gold Tiger Eye has a shimmering cat's-eye effect and is a yellow-gold banded stone. Reiki courses state that Gold Tiger Eye acts as a protector stone and can help with energy, grounding, material issues, and other spiritual matters.

Hematite is opaque and appears black. It is thick and heavy, and has a metallic shine. Many believe that Hematite can have relationships with destiny and predict future events.

Red Jasper Reiki crystal also comes in transparent and dark Terracotta. Red jasper helps to identify what is and not. It also inspires creativity.

Rose Quartz is pinkish and translucent. It is a calm stone with properties of warmth, gentleness, reconciliation, and warmth. It is great for learning all about female reproductive anatomy.

Snowflake Obisdian, which is a crystal of black with white dots, can also be used as a Reiki crystal. This pillar will help you clear any blocks and guide you in the correct direction. It can also be used to motivate people and help them recognize their potential.

Snow Quartz, a black, crystalline, rock. This Reiki crystal is well-known for its ability to cleanse the mind and promote rejuvenation.

Sodalite is a black, transparent rock that often contains a white vein. Reiki teaches that sodalite can make you feel young, give happiness, and lift your heart.

Unakite can be described as a pale green Reiki stone and is colored with salmon. It is known to harmonize energy, align it, and combine it. It's good. This allows for stability and can even resolve conflicts.

These are just a handful of the many Reiki crystal miracles described in Reiki classes. Reiki crystals can be fun. However, they will not cause harm if they aren't given to others. Reiki crystals will disappear if used in Reiki. They don't need to feel angry. Rock Reiki crystals!

What is Spiritual Health Coach?

Perhaps you've read about Spiritual Health Coaching. You will find answers to your questions from a spiritual coach in this book.

What is coaching spirituality and what does it mean?

You can find the answers to your spiritual questions and concerns by working with a certified Spiritual Health Coach. The Spiritual Health Coach will ask specific questions and provide a safe place for you to seek out answers. Because you already have all the answers, the Spiritual Wellness Coach only provides the resources necessary to seek them out.

It's as simple as that. Are you more likely than anyone else to take your advice? It's impossible to know the entire story.

What questions should a Spiritual Health Counselor ask?

This question was asked of me by both my family members and potential customers. Many people are asking what questions a Spiritual Health Coach should address, as Spiritual Health Coaching does not seem to be as common as some other types of coaching (e.g. job coaching, life coaching), Are you ready to take the next step in your spiritual journey? What is the right path for me spiritually? I don't know how to start but I do believe that I would like to communicate with a higher power. What's stopping me from moving forward in my spiritual development? A good idea is to talk to an SHC if you are having trouble with any aspect of your spirituality.

The SHC cannot deal with your physical and mental health problems, as well as legal issues. Spiritual wellness coaches are not qualified to diagnose any illness, or make recommendations in fields where they aren't certified.

Is it legal to provide information to SHC?

Spiritual Health Coaches are bound to keep your information confidential and strictly confidential. Your SHC should send you a confidentiality certificate before coaching sessions can begin. It makes sure that you are clear that any information you give the coach is confidential.

What can I anticipate and how long is that session?

This will depend on the Spiritual Coach you speak to. Sessions can either be held in person or over the phone, but most sessions are conducted by phone due not to distance. Coaches can alter the length of the sessions. Each mine takes between 40 minutes and an hour. This is because the consumer is assured that they feel that they have made significant progress on the subject, and that the session will end with an abrupt halt. Most spiritual coaches offer a free course in which you can learn more about your issues (and vice versa). You can view this as an intake meeting. This can be a good time to ask your future SHC questions. You may request a referral to another coach if Spiritual Health Coaching is not for you. Please note that the coach has the right to determine if a potential customer is a good fit and can refer you another instructor.

What happens during a session will depend on what the SHC decides. Below is a description of what I do during a session.

Unless something is relevant from the last session, I prefer learning about the successes and issues of my client throughout the week. Then, we'll discuss the "homework", you were given. Homework often involves reviewing questions and answering from the previous session. With a question and answers dialog, we can then join the work of the coaching sessions and gain insight and understanding into the areas you want to explore regarding spirituality.

Spiritual Health

There are various requirements at different levels. For instance, there are people within the realm that can find such things, like ourselves, and who need to improve the way they live. Others have more success rates because they are more likely to inherit their behavior from less intelligent creatures. Your interaction with your colleagues does not rank higher than your personal contact.

This is how we look at life and consider what it is like to not have the things that we have been given. As you can imagine, we are fortunate in comparison to other real plains. However, not all of us are as fortunate as those who live in more privileged areas.

It's just like that for us.

You can have different levels of what you call spiritual health in your life. Some of you may feel safe, regardless what your beliefs are, while others might be very sick and require some help.

It's just like that with us.

You can improve yourself by doing the same things that we do for others. We believe that you need a higher level of sense. We are seeking answers to the mystery surrounding all the plains and creation. We are trying to find ways to improve in many areas. One discipline involves spinning a circle and choosing an area. We attempt to pinpoint the point each time the globe turns.

As you can see, our exercises are vital.

You do something a little unusual, because you almost always need to return to your inner man. Your meditation and prayer, or yoga. These practices are beneficial and will allow you to see beyond your current reality.

Your well-being is about recognizing all the ways you have disconnected yourself from the world you live in. Understanding that you are an individual with a soul means that you should care about your path because that will impact the direction of the soul.

Then, we'll offer some advice. That is what we want.

You must decide first. Act kindly.

First, you need to agree that every action you take will benefit yourself and everyone in your immediate vicinity.

A second thing you must do is pay attention to the people close to you. This could be your wife, husband or children.

Third, get rid of all doubts and fears. It is never over if you are fully present in the moment.

When you are feeling confused, it is important to not give up. You should assume that these values have been acquired by living as mature adults. It is also a strength that certainty offers.

This means that we are aware of what is happening and move forward. It is a sign that your experience has tested you. And individual behavior is what determines how you perceive the world.

What would it be like to take with you, if you were gone and dead? Only one thing can you take with your, which is your eternal spirit or your mind or consciousness.

What does spirituality look like? If you are able to see the truth of the universe and your own existence without doubt. You can recognize the existence of other types or levels of existence.

Keep this in mind as you approach your day. You will find your soul living in the whole world.

The thing that we want in our spheres is what they see. To be friends with each other is our reward.

Take the time to see now. Be confident in your ability to face the world with your whole heart and let your emotions guide you. A real understanding of your identity and where you're going will help you set goals. All the things you see in your world have been achieved because they were planted as seeds. Only love and faith can make your life a reality.

You are part a greater real estate than you realize.

How can you be sure you have achieved your goals even if you're not there yet? Some people will grasp their purpose and then move on to fulfill it. Others will not understand. It must be something that you asked for before you were born. It is possible to get what you ask for. While it is wonderful to wish, you cannot make anything. It's important to be able to see what has been given. This will make you happy because you won't be in need.

What you attract is what it has already been. You can choose to not act or speak, or you may even be unable to recognize that it is yours. You can manifest an interest once you find what you were looking for. If you look within, you will find this out. This will help you to see your true self. When you pray, keep your eyes on the present moment.

Chapter 6: Seven Chakras Overview

It is impossible to begin a discussion on crystal healing without a basic understanding about the chakras. These three principles are fundamental to all of life.

1. The principle behind energy

2. The principle and practice of duality

3. The principle of equilibrium

The principle of Energy states that everything, from the air we breathe to the ground where we stand, has its own unique energy. This energy is in constant circulation, and it is what makes all activity possible. It is found in the elemental elements of earth (Prithvi), space (Akasha), fire(Tejas), water (Jala), and fire (Tejas).

This energy is also known as Prana. This energy or force is likened with a thread, which when cut causes death and decay. It is important to understand the principle duality and balance in order to understand Prana's ability to sustain life. The principle o duality, also called the principle o polarity is a requirement that every positive action or condition must have a counter action. Physics has its own version. The principle states that "for every action, the opposite reaction" means that everything should have an opposite. This is why everything has pairs: male and female, good or bad, push or pull, life and demise, yin yang.

Only in the midst this polarity can balance be found. The graphic representations, yin and Yang, show how balance can be found in the midst. The two halves, the yin or white and the yang or black, are halves of a complete circle. The full circle is the life force, while the halves represent the polar forces. The only thing that can sustain all life is the union of these polar energies, with the exception of exceptional cases of higher consciousness. This explanation can be used as a reason for the four seasons that feature two periods (spring/summer) of plenty, beauty and activity, while two periods (fall/winter) are of no, starkness, rest and death.

The principle o balance states that the forces must be in harmony. They should not have too much of one or too few of each other, a Goldilocks state of "just right" or "middle". Prana is energy for all of life. It operates on the principle duality and polarity. This is why breathing is more than a one-time action. It involves two parts: inhaling, and exhaling. It would be impossible to breathe if you keep inhaling and not exhaling. If we inhale and exhale, it would be exactly the same. To ensure that the threads of life are held taut it must be fixed to the poles inhaling/exhaling. Here it is important that Prana not only refers to the air that we inhale or exhale but is also the force that controls all aspects of our body, including breathing.

Man is made up of seven bodies. Some schools of thinking divide these bodies into the spiritual, subtle and physical. Harmony between all these bodies is essential for life to continue unaffected.

The Chakras are a collection energy points at different points within the body. It is often represented as a spinning wheel, or disc. Each chakra has its own point of action in the body.

Although we may say that the fifth chakra is located at glabella it doesn't guarantee we will see it. We won't see any chakras if someone is cut open. The chakras, which are not part our physical bodies, are part the subtle body. There are seven different chakras. The fourth chakra, which is also called the only human chakra, is often used to denote that it is what separates humans from animals.

Man is often referred either to as a god who is in disarray (or a god who is being made). This means that the disarray is what makes man a man. In the absence this disarray, he can attain a godlike standing. To achieve a godlike status, one must climb from within the first chakra (Muladhara), all the way to the top of seventh chakra (Sahaswara). However, the climb can be daunting and is filled with setbacks and failures. In the pursuit of Sahaswara, enlightenment and conquering that disarray, we discover about the chakras.

There are seven chakras.

1. Muladhara, or the root chakra

2. Svadhisthana, or the sacral chakra.

3. Manipura: The solar plexus Chakra, Manipura

4. Anahata, The Heart Chakra

5. Vishuddha is the throat chakra

6. Ajna, third eye chakra

7. Sahaswara, The Crown Chakra

Muladhara (The Root Chakra).

This is the primary chakra. It represents stability and the need to survive. Saturn and Earth both influence the first chakra. They represent the need for stability and survival. This chakra can be found at the base or the perineum of the spine. Muladhara people are most concerned about their food and survival.

Food is more than food. It can also be money, wealth, or anything that allows us to survive. A person who operates at the chakra level is just like an animal. He is constantly obsessed with how to acquire more food, and even though he has enough, it does not feel sufficient.

Muladhara's motto, "survival is the best," is his motto. He will do everything to preserve his food or other means of survival. He is always on fight or flight mode. To exist at the level of the chakra is the greatest disservice one could do to himself.

Svadhisthana - The Sacral Chakra

This chakra is the second and second. It is located in sacral plexus. This chakra refers the fluid energy of creativity, sex, and is influenced by changing energies like water, Pluto, and moon. This is a yin energy, which is stronger in women. The energy of the second Chakra is what provides us with creativity and guides all our sexual affairs.

Muladhara who is self-centered and seeks to make his own way in life through sex, Muladhara takes and attempts to find his place. Svadhisthana gives, and tries hard to establish roots. Muladhara doesn't have this ability, so Svadhisthana is a higher level than Muladhara. This chakra is often called "chakra of Life" and is closely associated with sex. Sex is what produces life and Jala (water), is what is at the root of all things.

Anybody who can channel this powerful sexual energy is on the right track to greatness. This chakra should not be the only place where divinity can be found.

Manipura (The Solar Plexus Chakra).

This is the third chakra, and the last among the animal Chakras. It is located at solar plexus. It is a fiery energy chakra and is governed by the energies of fire, the sun, or mars. It is often called the "chakra of the personality" because it is a yang (or masculine) chakra. Manipura allows you to see yourself as a whole, without relying on external factors.

Manipura regulates confidence and esteem. When it becomes imbalanced, it can result in excessive ego and pride as well as low self-esteem. As with everything else in the universe, ego can only be bad when there are surpluses or deficits. Manipura man views himself as the sun. Bright, glorious, all-powerful. Notable. He believes everyone should revolve around his world. He is a type A personality, who is a choleric.

The creative and imaginative power of Svadhisthana is translated into action by the fiery Manipura. If left uncontrolled, the Manipura's attractive, powerful, and endearing man can quickly turn to a harsh, abrasive.

Anahata, The Heart Chakra

This chakra is also the fourth and final human chakra. It is said that below the hearts man is an animal and above them God becomes God. However, it is at the heart that man is man. This chakra is affected by Venus and serves as a transition from the wild to the ethereal. Anahata, the yin energies of love, is pure love that expects nothing back. Anahata is not a erotic, obsessive, or conditional type of love. Instead, Anahata promotes self-suffering and unconditional love.

This is the place where love can be self-effacingly altruistic. This love is like agape, and we can learn to love as the Maker loves. Anahata's seat is his physical heart.

Vishuddha - The Throat Chakra

This is also the fifth chakra. This is the point where man begins to journey into the divine. Mercury and Jupiter rule this chakra. It is associated with the search for the truth and the voicing it at all costs. This is why the chakra's location is the throat.

Vishuddha literally means purity. This is the first step toward reclaiming that pure, pristine part within you that has been hidden in filth and darkness so long. This chakra is the key to being persuasive and charismatic. Vishudha not only helps us make the truth a beacon dispelling ignorance and darkness but also gives words, thoughts, affirmations, and words a certain power. Vishudha will deliver you to nirvana through helping you establish a better link channel between your intrinsic, and extrinsic realms.

Ajna is the Third Eye Chakra

This is the sixth chakra, the second divine chakra. It is influenced and located between the eyebrows, at the glabella. This chakra is for introspection. Introspection, intuition and deep thought. Because it can clairvoyance, the Ajna Man's life is filled with concurrent feelings of déjà vu.

He is introspective, and learns how to trust his sixth sense. This chakra is often called sixth sense chakra. Ajna is a powerful energy that increases Svadhisthana. It also allows you to have many innovative ideas. The need for duality disappears at this point. You can transcend and no longer be affected by the elements. You can see it and transcend time and place.

Sahaswara (The Crown Chakra).

This is the seventh, last, and third divine chakra. It is also the endpoint, the centre of energy and the point where all things are at rest. Its physical location can be found at the crown on the head. Uranus influences it. Sahaswara is where enlightenment occurs and we reach nirvana.

We become like the thousand-petaled lotus pushing through the dirt and mud to enjoy the sun. We learn that you can only be truly wise if you admit to your ignorance.

So why is chakras so important, other than enlightenment? If the chakras are balanced, they can help us strengthen our connection with the source of everything. They can be understood, accepted, and balanced. It will help us gain mastery over our mind and self, as well as liberate and release our most negative traits. This will greatly improve interpersonal relationships and intrapersonal relationships. This delicate balance is what opens up the realm of crystal heal.

Chapter 7: How To Choose Your Crystals

When selecting your crystals, you should take into account the price, the problem you are trying to solve and the chakra that you want to balance. However, most often it is the crystal who chooses you. It is best to shop in person for crystals and not online.

A crystal is like an universal messenger who comes into your life to help you get on the right track, balance your energies, emotions and actions, help you learn valuable lessons and help make you the best version possible. Crystals can have different energies which appeal to different people. A strong influx of energies would hit you when you walk into any crystal shop. But, certain energies of specific crystals might resonate more strongly with you. This is a strange connection that you might have with the mineral kingdom. You'd probably be smiling right about now.

A crystal can be described as a good friend. When you first meet them, you instantly feel connected and like you've known them forever. It is important to always have such a stone with you, in order for it to be able to access your energy and vibrations.

Begin with one crystal, and then see what effect it has on your body and energy. Nature has provided us with a variety of crystals. Below you will find a selection of the most popular crystals as well their gifts and the elemental chakras and signs they correspond with.

Clear Quartz

This clear, colorless, crystal is associated with the crown chakra (Sahaswara), as well as the sun. But, generally speaking, this jacks-of-all-trades stone helps to open all the chakras, Muladhara to Sahaswara. It is known to have amazing curative powers and can amplify energy and thought. It regulates, awakens, stores, releases and amplifies the energies of all other crystals. It can simply do the work of any other crystal if you ask it.

All that is required to make the crystal clear with your thoughts is to place your own thoughts into it. It removes any negative energy and neutralizes the background radiation. It balances, organizes and revitalizes the mental, physical, and spiritual levels. It is a powerful healing stone and can help with any condition.

It cleanses and revitalizes the organs, and the subtle body. It removes negative energy from the soul and reconnects the physical and mental dimensions. It is also related to the Crown Chakra. It improves psychic abilities, memory, clarity, thinking, and awareness. It aids us in accessing our spiritual guide. This facilitates and speeds the discovery and realization of our higher self.

It restores balance to the body and heals immune system problems. It harmonizes the chakras, Muladhara and Sahaswara. This keeps the subtle body in peace. If you cannot afford to purchase any additional stones, or you wish to only work with one stone at a time it is better to use this or carnelian.

CARNELIAN

The element of fire corresponds with Muladhara Manipura and Svadhisthana. It can add zest to your life and increase sexual energy.

It can help you get rid of procrastination and overwhelm negativity. It will also boost your vital energy and confidence. Carnelian stimulates creativity, physical power, and compassion.

Lapis Lazuli

It is available in different shades. It helps you to balance Ajna or Vishuddha. It helps you see the truth and speaks it. It is often associated with Taurus as well as Sagittarius. It guards against psychic attacks. The element water is what makes it so relaxing and gives you deep peace.

It can bring harmony and deepen your understanding of yourself. It allows you to express your inner self, exposes inner truths and provides immortality, honesty, compassion, as well as the ability to show compassion.

It increases objectivity, clarity, and creativity. Lapis Lazuli creates bonds that allow for the better expression and expression of emotions. It strengthens the immune system and helps to eliminate vertigo, insomnia, depression, and blood pressure. It has a strong connection to the fifth, sixth, and seventh chakras. It also benefits the nervous and respiratory systems, throats, vocal chords, and thyroid. It strengthens the bone and thymus.

Tiger's Eye

It corresponds both to the Sacral Chakra (Muladhara), as well as the Solar Plexus Chakra (Manipura), so you're not surprised that the elements it corresponds too are fire and earth. This stone of protection can double as a luck charm. It helps to clear the mind by bringing clarity and intuition.

It is especially useful for curing psychosomatic illness, dispelling fear or anxiety, and understanding one's personal needs and how they influence others. Tiger's eyes stabilize mood swings and instills self-confidence, willpower, purposefulness, courage, self-confidence, and tension. They also restore equilibrium to the yin/yang energies and strengthen the emotional body.

Tiger's eyes are effective in treating eye, throat, reproductive and other ailments. They also detoxify, soothe pain, and help with broken bones, scoliosis, strengthening the spine, and helping to heal scoliosis.

AMETHYST

This stone can be found in various shades of purple. Amethyst increases your ability to perceive by clearing the third eye. Watching too many TV programs, reading articles online or interacting with people who are negative can lead to the third eye becoming cluttered. This crystal helps to maintain the functioning of the pineal & pituitary glands.

Ajna also corresponds to Sahaswara. They use it to activate the crown chakra and clear it. It is the February birthstone. It corresponds with the zodiacs Virgo. Its elements are water and air.

Amethyst comes in a range of colors, from a slight pinkish violet to light grey purple. All shades have their own properties. Protective stone amethyst that protects against psychic attacks, transforms energy to love, and protects against all kinds of harm and ill wishes.

Amethyst represents spirituality and intuition. It provides stability, strength and inner calm. It's great for meditation and improving your intuition. Amethyst is an excellent stress-reliever and natural tranquilizer. It calms tension and irritability and balances mood swings. The stone is said to bring an increase in feelings of sadness, sorrow, and negativity.

It has strong cleansing and healing properties and promotes sobriety. It can calm and stimulate the mind to help you be more focused. It increases your retention and self-motivation. Also, it gives you a sense of clarity that helps you remember and interpret your dreams.

Amethyst can help with insomnia by bringing calmness to the body. If you suffer from insomnia, put amethyst in your pillowcase and add a few drops or lavender oil. The warmth and energy of amethyst increases selflessness as well as spiritual wisdom. It increases hormone production by correcting disorders of the endocrinology system. It improves the immune system and reduces pain. This helps fight against rapidly growing cancer cells.

It can destroy malignant tumours and promote tissue regeneration. It clarifies the blood and reduces stress-related pain. It can also be used to treat auditory conditions and respiratory diseases.

Rose Quartz

It is associated to Anahata Chakra and its Zodiacs are Taurus & Libra. Its elements are water and earth. Its most popular color is rose-pink. It is the stone for unconditional and universal love. It eases conflict, releases the pain that comes with relationships, and promotes love. The feeling of being protected and loved when wearing or carrying it is similar to feeling in the mother's womb.

Rose quartz makes us feel loved and warms our hearts. It encourages true, unconditional, genuine, and sincere love. It is a purifier of the heart, promoting love, self-love. friendship, emotional healing, peace and calmness. It is a comforting and hopeful tool in times of loss. It is a positive and encouraging tool that encourages forgiving (of oneself and of others), trust, acceptance, forgiveness, and lets go of negative emotional attachments.

Rose quartz is excellent for those times when you feel alone or in need to have more love, comfort, affection, and support. Rose quartz has been worn by people who reported feeling the warm embrace and nature's love. It can reduce stress and tension. It allows us express emotions such as love, compassion, happiness, and joy easily and effectively. Rose quartz can help protect you from negative influences in your environment, strengthen your heart and improve your cardiovascular system.

It can also speed up recovery, stabilize blood pressure, treat chest and lung problems and the kidney and adrenal cells. It's a great energy supplement for patients with leukemia. It can improve fertility, protect the mother and baby during pregnancy and prevent miscarriage. The yoni eggs form of this crystal strengthens the pelvic floor muscles. This crystal makes sex more enjoyable and improves the relationship between you and your partner. To relieve headaches, eczema or migraines, use a rose quartz pointed and rose oil to massage the temples.

Moss Agate

It has the element earth and the zodiac Virgo. It corresponds to both the sacral and heart chakras. It is the stone of new beginnings, and blank slates. It revitalizes the spirit, helps you get rid of past mistakes, and makes it possible to see things in a whole new way. It calms inflammation and reduces sensitivity. It will make your financial life easier and increase self-esteem. It improves interpersonal and intrapersonal connections and strengthens the wearer.

The positive effects of Moss agate are a refreshing boost to creativity, especially when one is having a tough time finding creative inspiration. It promotes self expression through your writing and creative activities. This stone is a good choice for those who are struggling with depression or despair. It also helps improve communication and foster trust.

Moss agate not only helps to calm inflammation and cure ailments of digestion and excretory, but it also improves the immune system's performance. It helps to reduce the pains of childbirth and stabilizes serum glucose.

Black Tourmaline

It helps stabilize the root chakra. It helps to stabilize the root chakra. We can get so focused on our survival in life that we barely take a moment to appreciate all that life offers. This stone can help us to have that pause. It allows us to truly experience all the tastes and experiences of life. Black tourmaline will help you to end bad habits and dangerous ideas. This makes your aura more positive and draws out all negativity you might have seen or harbored from others. It's especially beneficial for empaths that make the pain of others theirs.

AQUAMARINE

It corresponds the Vishuddha chakra, the throat chakra. This is the stone for clarity and purification. It is a stone of clarity and purification. This stone is great for sensitive people, as it can calm riotous emotions and promote self-courage. It helps heal fifth chakra imbalances. It also strengthens the thyroid, liver, pituitary, and throat glands. It is good for all the chakras, but it's especially good for the throat chakra.

CITRINE

This stone corresponds Manipura (the third chakra). This stone takes its energy from the sun's fiery power. It is a cheerful stone that gives you joy, courage, hope and warmth. It is believed that it holds the energy of sun. Manipura can be opened and activated from this stone. This will allow us to discover who we are and improve our self-esteem, self expression, and creativity.

Citrine is the stone associated with success, abundance, prosperity. It is therefore a vital stone for anyone experiencing financial hardship. It can help you achieve your dreams, by harnessing the positive energies of the sun. Citrine is a powerful, cleansing, and rejuvenating stone that awakens mind, body, soul.

For healing, it protects your digestive organs and the liver, reduces infection, inflammation, promotes tissue regeneration, detoxification, and good circulation. Citrine stimulates the crown, as well as energizing the base chakra.

FLUORITE

This dark purple rock is the stone that brings stability, insight, and understanding. Like the clear quartz fluorite aids in opening and awakening third eye chakra. It is also known to promote focus, intuition and stability as well as free-thinking, clear thinking, and clarity. Fluorite acts as a protector stone and draws away negative thoughts, stress, worry and anxiety.

It can also cleanse and clarify blood and the whole body. It is also believed to strengthen bones, teeth, and aid in emotional and psychological trauma. It helps to prevent and treat a variety of illnesses, from the common cold and flus to heart conditions.

AVENTURINE

This stone gives you a calm and easy-going attitude towards life. Aventurine is a heart chakra activator, protector and clearer. It helps to balance the energies yin/yang and attracts joy, happiness, emotional and mental calmness and positivity into your life. It supports the well-being of our physical, psychological, and spiritual bodies.

This crystal will make you more passionate about your life, your creative activities, and your relationships. It promotes empathy and motivation. It calms anger and provides independence. It stimulates your mind and gets one creative juices flowing. It also helps to heal your heart chakra.

It prevents pollution from entering the body, supports the formation and healing broken bones, calms migraines, stabilizes blood pressure, cholesterol levels, and protects against other environmental pollutants. It is also known to reduce anxiety, fear, stress, and promote peaceful sleep.

Red Jasper

Muladhara, also known as the root chakra, corresponds to this warm redstone. It aids in balancing our lives and keeping us grounded. Red Jasper supports and encourages stress relief by warming and activating the soul.

It helps you take control of your own life and encourages you not to give up. This stone treats disorders related to digestion and blood circulation. Red Jasper can also help to balance the throat chakra.

LABORITE

This stone works in all areas of your mind and body. It is excellent for meditation because it increases the energy flow through our body.

It enhances the brightness and quality of your aura, stimulates rational thought and intuition, and raises consciousness. This is the key to making our dreams and goals a reality.

You can also use this stone to communicate the intention of others. It is known to help balance hormones and emotions, stabilize blood pressure, and treat brain and optical disorders. It is especially helpful for the crown chakra, heart chakra, third eye chakra, and third eye chakra.

HEMATITE

This is a metallic heavy stone and an iron mine. It is excellent for working with the first chakra. It helps with sleep problems, promotes relaxation, and fights nightmares.

It can be placed under your pillow or on your bedside table. It is full with tamasic energetic, which can help you relax, calm down, and find peace in all spheres of life.

Other useful stones

Amber purifies the system, treats digestive ailments, activates third chakra and gives self-confidence, self-esteem and self-worth.

Black Obsidian activates your root chakra and connects you more strongly to the steady, solid energy of the Earth.

Bloodstone balances each elemental chakra and opens our hearts and minds to the warmth, blessings, and power of the fourth.

Corals enhance emotions and vibratory energy of the heart chakra.

Sapphire is a tranquilizer that fills the heart and mind. It restores balance and stability by anchoring and sustaining us.

Garnet stimulates your root chakra (Muladhara), which helps to eliminate all negative energy.

Kyanite instantly activates, aligns and balances each of the seven chakras.

Emeralds are antidepressants that can be viewed as crystalline. They promote peaceful sleep and restful sleep.

Malachite stimulates your heart chakra. It makes you more open to both internal and external love, friendships, and peace. It opens the throat chakra. This allows us not only to speak the truth but also to live life in the world around us.

Moonstone helps to detoxify and restore balance to all the chakras.

Diamonds enhance prosperity and promote clarity of thought.

Turquoise activates and opens the throat chakra. This improves interpersonal and intrapersonal communication. It also enhances the energies in the other six chakras.

Chapter 8: Crystals

"In a crystal we have clear evidence for a formative principle of life. And although we cannot understand everything about the life of a cristal, it is still an alive being."

Nikola Tesla

Our entire body system is made up of energy. Energy comes in many densities and patterns. Even thoughts and emotions can have energy and densities that are their own and which are connected to the physical body. We experience good health when these patterns of energy are harmonious and balanced. But, these energy patterns may be disrupted by certain factors that are both controllable but uncontrollable. This can lead to illnesses. These can range anywhere from headaches and serious diseases.

Crystals are the strongest form of matter, because they were formed over many years at a distance far beneath the Earth. The Greek roots for the word "crystal", which means "ice", are Greek. The reason is that the ancient Greeks believed crystals were water that had frozen to a point at which it would never again become liquid. Crystals form in earth's crust after millions of years of high pressure and heat. Each step of crystal formation is rich in energy.

The crystal journey begins beneath the planet's surface, where magma circulates and degrades materials to make crystallization possible. Crystallization occurs when layers in the earth's core fracture, allowing hot gases and liquids to push toward the surface.

Additional to water, elements such oxygen, sodium iron, potassium, magnesium, and iron are also present. They combine and dissolve with elements that are pushed to the top. Crystal formation occurs when the mixture rises and passes through lower-active layers of rock.

Crystallization depends on environmental conditions and available forms of elements. The environment and available formative elements have a significant impact on crystal growth. These include temperature, time, pressure, light, pressure, time and distance. Tesla is right to say that crystals are living beings and can work with the energy field of the body to absorb, move, change, or diffuse energy.

The vibration levels of crystals depend on their composition and colors. Each crystal vibrates at its own frequency, much like individual cells within the human body. Crystals, just like the chakras, work by naturally focusing, magnifying, and equalizing the body's innate energies.

They can be used to reduce pain and facilitate desired changes in your life. Because crystals vibrate with our vibration, when they come into contact with us, we feel their vibration. These crystals are useful for many purposes, including crystals in calculators and clocks as well as crystals used in smartphones, cell phones and lasers for microscopic surgeries. The body's natural rhythm can be restored by using crystal energy.

Crystal Healing - Truth Or Hoax?

Crystal healing is simply a way to use crystals to heal your mental, physical, and spiritual ailments. You can do this by either placing the crystals on the areas where you feel or believe the pain is, or by using a grid to place the crystals under your pillow in places that you spend most your time.

By using patterns, combinations of stones can be used to enhance, supplement and complement their individual properties. You will feel reconnected to yourself and the earth by restoring energy flow through your meridians, energy centers, and brain activity.

Healing is not performed at the conscious level. It takes place at the subconscious levels. Crystals are able to help you tap into the subconscious mind and heal. They work as a subconscious reminder, reminding your body, emotions, or spirit man that it is time to get back in the game. They can also affect the external environment in your favor. The foundation of crystal healing is the belief in crystals having unique energetic vibrations. These vibrations can balance the vibrations of our bodies, and help us get rid of sickness.

Over the centuries, precious stones and crystals have been used as healing tools to improve physical, mental, and spiritual wellbeing. People of old, shamans, and other healers must have known that crystals could interact with the energy fields of the human body to create subtle but perceptible energy shifts.

Royals have worn a variety of crystals throughout history. They used them to decorate their crowns as jewelry, thrones and shields. It is interesting that having a particular crystal in your crown activates your crown chakra. For instance, a necklace over your heart could activate and activate your heart chakra. Rings could stimulate energy flow through you meridians while earrings would stimulate our reflexes.

This arrangement makes it seem as if jewelry was more than just adornments. It connects different healing stones to different energy points on your body. Dr. Rob Lavinsky a leading expert in crystal and minerals, stated:

"When you speak of feeling the power in the stone, what are you feeling? Your body's electric field (or what some people call the aura), going into the crystal. Then you will feel a kind of biofeedback loop. You may also see the reflection of your energies through the crystal. Crystals are capable of refracting, reflecting, and conducting energy back to you ..."

People believe crystals incite healing because they balance and align our chakras (which are basically energies) by activating them, opening them or closing. Crystal healing is basically about correcting imbalances in energy. A crystal can be used to provide the same energy as the energy that caused the problem.

Alternative medicine dates back thousands of years to ancient civilizations like Egypt. The ancients had a great deal of knowledge about crystals and the healing properties they could provide, so they included them in nearly all of life's activities. To help guide their souls into the afterlife, the ancient Egyptians buried their victims with a piece if quartz on each forehead. They also used crystals for healing elixirs.

Ancient Egyptian belly-dancers were known to have worn ruby stones on the belly buttons. It was believed this enhanced their sexuality and increased their creativity. It was also believed that wearing a necklace with a pendant of crystals over your heart will attract love. A forehead crown was also worn to stimulate your third eye. To balance their yin yang energies, the Pharaohs carried copper cylinders as well as zinc cylinders. Chrysolite was used in Egypt to fight severe nightmares, and exorcise evil spirits.

Clear quartz crystals were thought to be the heart of dragons and represented wisdom and power by the ancient Japanese. Hematite can be described as an iron ore. Aries is the Greek god of war. Crushed hematite was believed to give the Greeks invincibility and helped them get ready for battle. Hematite is actually derived form the Greek word Heme, which means blood. This is due to the reddish-tinged crystals get when they undergo oxidation. Amethyst, however, is the opposite and means "not drunken". It was worn as an amulet in order to prevent hangovers and inebriation.

Crystals were used to attract and treat diseases in ancient Rome. They were also used to enhance health and provide protection during battle. The ancient Romans also wore crystal amulets that they believed brought peace.

India's sacred texts spoke out about crystals being used as a method of treating diseases, mental illnesses, and other conditions. Ayurveda in India, another form of wellbeing, recognizes the healing potential of crystals for hundreds years.

The Mayans as well as the Sumerians aren't left out, since they all understood the metaphysical properties of crystals for healing and balance at emotional, mental, physical and spiritual levels. These civilizations used crystals as a way to diagnose and cure diseases. In some accounts, Incas believed that some stones (emeralds), were so valuable that they would rather pay the eternal price than reveal the locations of their mines to their enemies.

Jade is believed to have spiritual significance in China. Jade was recognized as a kidney heal stone by both the ancient South American cultures and Chinese. Quartz crystal spheres were believed to be objects that had great holy spiritual powers. They could be used to help attain enlightenment in Tibet. This is not far off the truth, since it aids in activating third eye chakra and crown chakras. Both of these are essential for man to rise above ignorance and attain the highest level of awakening.

Crystal healing offers many advantages. It is safe and painless. You are not using modern medicine's side effects. Instead, you are using an attractive, nontoxic gift that nature gives to help remove any negative emotions, diseases, or ailments. The crystal will replace these with its warm, glowing energy. Crystals work together, and unlike drugs that sometimes clash with one another, they are always in harmony. Clear quartz can provide many benefits and won't interfere at all with the gifts your amethyst crystals and hematite.

There has been much debate about crystal healing's efficacy. Many believe it is not scientifically supported or has the same route of action as regular drugs. Chris French is a prominent expert on paranormal psychology and conducted a study of the healing potential of crystals. He gave people different crystals and asked them to relax and to meditate, then primed them with what they were expecting to feel.

These sensations were triggered by a lot of crystals. But, even though some of those crystals were false placebos (fakes), those holding them still felt the healing vibrations. But what scientists might call "pilloids", we call it intention. Take it as this: If you suffer from headaches, you will search for an anti-inflammatory drug and then take it. Why? Because you believe aspirin will ease the headache. Crystal healing works because of your belief and intention. It is one thing to believe and two things to act. There is a good chance that you won't believe they are effective.

Crystal healing can actually be studied. Energy is everywhere. Energy is everywhere. Everything we see, from solid objects like a sofa to fragile things like hair strands, are energy vibrations. While scientists have found ways to use crystals to make computers, timepieces and other parts for smartphones and some drugs, they have not yet discredited their use of crystals in healing.

Consider a crystal as a magnet. It attracts and repels negative vibrations with its energy, which can bring you feelings such as peace, calmness, and well-being. Marcel Vogel is an IBM scientist. He was one of the few people to conduct scientific experiments to verify the effectiveness of crystals. Vogel noticed crystals changing shape under a microscope while studying how they were grown. Vogel linked this change in form to the constant assembly, disassembling and reassembling fundamental bonds between the crystals' molecules.

His experiments with quartz crystals showed that crystals can also store thoughts and intention in the same manner as tapes do sound, thanks to the use of magnetic energy.

Crystals basically work by:

* Enhance the positive vibrations you send out

* Shifting low frequencies of illness. Sickness is found in low frequencies of vibrations. You can vibrate at a higher level and diseases won't be

able to get to you. This is what I have discussed in my book Chakra healing. You can vibrate at a higher frequency without any diseases by using crystals.

* To help us establish and reestablish our connection with Mother Earth's healing powers and to her.

You must set an intention to get a crystal working before you can make it work. Imagine holding the crystal in one's hand, and feeling it radiate warmth. Now, create your intention. First, identify the areas in which you need to be more positive. This will also help you to determine which combinations or stones to choose. Do you feel that your creative life, financial health, relationships, or social life could use a boost?

After you have identified the problem, ask yourself what is most important and which problem are you trying to solve first. Crystals can be so captivating and star-studded, and it is easy to lose track of what is most important. But you must prioritize and follow a "divide, conquer" approach.

It is essential to identify the area of your life that needs immediate attention. After this, you can begin working on other areas. As you get more comfortable with the energies of the crystal, the next areas will become easier. Once you have decided on the area that you want to work on, be specific about your goals. Be specific about your goals, the timeframe you would like them to take place and the reasons you believe they are important.

Consider this: If I had a piece o rose quartz (a stone of love), and I pictured a bright, shining light through it, I would set my intention accordingly.

I am filled up with light and love. This connects me with my higher self, the pure and highest self, which is closest to the divine. I command this rose quartz, to hold my intentions for pure and true love. I promise to love and be loved. I will be able to accept and love myself regardless of my flaws. I realize that I deserve love. So, as I love today and in the future, I will be open for love. I won't let past hurts stop me loving my mother and her gifts. I will learn to love myself unconditionally and the people around me. This would make me a better human being and draw me closer towards the source and maker of everything. I open my heart and mind to healthy love, strong friends, and peace. I have earned them. We are grateful for your support of this intention. Thank you for setting it all in motion and making it a reality. We are so grateful that you made it possible.

After repeating these words, you can blow on the crystal 3 times. The crystal will absorb your intentions, work on them and help you reach your goals. The three-times you thank the crystal, it has already made your intentions a reality.

Crystal healing is not magic. But there are others who believe crystals work. They will get crystals, make intentions, and wait for them to work. They blame the crystals when they fail to get what they want. Crystals don't work that way. Crystals, vibrations at fundamental levels, can be used to shift your natural vibration and bring about a change.

We also found that healing requires action as well as belief. So, along with believing, you must work. Only then could the crystal perform well. It's impossible to be a solitary person and expect the rose quartz will deliver love to you via DHL. You have to be out there. You are the only thing rose quartz can do for you.

Chapter 9: Uses For Crystals

The healing powers of crystals are the focus of this book. But these crystals' healing abilities don't end there. Crystals can help you relax, improve your focus, and even prevent psychic attacks. They have been used to enhance the beauty, sexuality and spirituality of people.

I've discovered three major uses for crystals from my studies:

* Applications physical

* Pharmaceutical and medical applications

* Spiritual applications

Physical Purposes

Different crystals, including diamonds, sapphires rubies, quartzes and rubies, have been extremely useful in many of our domestic as well as industrial activities. Diamonds, we all know are the strongest natural objects. Diamonds are so strong that only one shard of diamond can be used to cut them. It is no surprise that bits of diamonds can be used to create industrial saws. These saws are used by jewelers as well as lapidary artisans for shaping ornamental gemstones, including sapphire and jade. Also, diamond crystals are used to make oil well drilling tools.

Timepieces can be made of precious stones, crystals, like ruby, quartz, and sapphire. Quartz controls the movement in all three hands. Rolex watches use a special type of sapphire to make their glass. Rolex watches do not tick, but sweep like other types of timepieces made from quartz crystals.

Pure quartz sand has been used to create integrated circuits, microelectronics as well as the silicon chip. Hard bearings in watches are made with rubies. Also, lasers of high intensity and minimal divergence can be made using rubies. These lasers can also be found in CD-players, telephones and some surveying equipment. Crystals can also serve as powering calculators, transistors (bulb filaments), solar cells, and LCD (Liquid Crystal Display).

It is also well-known that these crystals aid in communication. Carrying a topaz or aquamarine crystal will make it easier to communicate with others, improve your confidence, and avoid any misunderstandings.

The addition of crystals and stones such as garnet, carnelian ruby rose quartz, bloodstone and pink tourmaline to your sexual experience and relationships can make it more exciting. They work in a variety of ways. Tourmaline helps to lower inhibitions, while rose quartz boosts the levels of feel-good hormones like Oxytocin and Ruby. Research has shown that certain stones such as aventurine and moss agate can also help with financial recovery.

Crystals can also serve decorative and aesthetic purposes. They are the centerpiece of all necklaces, bracelets and rings. They can also decorate your home, shops, and restaurants.

Pharmacological and Medical Uses

Medical practitioners of the new age have discovered and confirmed the healing properties crystals have on various diseases and ailments. Amethyst is a remarkable crystal that can soothe migraines and stabilize blood sugar. The healing properties of carnelian, emeralds and sapphires have been proven to help in the relief of pains related to menstrual cramps. A lot of crystals, especially amethyst are known to alleviate nightmares and insomnia. They can also bring sweet dreams and restful sleeping when placed close to the sleeping area.

Spiritual Uses

This is where much has been done, especially by yogis or people seeking greater awareness. As stated earlier, man is composed of seven bodies. The spiritual body can be considered one of these seven. One of the seven bodily systems can go wrong, and it will affect six others. The care and wellbeing for each of these seven bodies should be prioritized.

Crystals aid in keeping the spiritual man healthy by activating, aligning and activating the chakras. This helps us avoid psychic and spiritual attacks and negative karma. It also helps us get closure from the past and calms the turbulent waters of emotions.

www.ingramcontent.com/pod-product-compliance
Lightning Source LLC
Chambersburg PA
CBHW050402120526
44590CB00015B/1788